Biliary Tract - Disease, Treatment, and Quality of Life

Edited by Qiang Yan

Published in London, United Kingdom

Biliary Tract - Disease, Treatment, and Quality of Life
http://dx.doi.org/10.5772/intechopen.1003471
Edited by Qiang Yan

Assistants to Editor: Zhenhua Tan and Jing Mao

Contributors
Alexander Sockell, Brian Gilchrist, Mohie El-Din Mostafa Madany, Petar Filev, Pratibha Vemulapalli, Prem Kurra, Qiang Yan, Sabina Więcek, Sotirov Dobromir Yordanov, Sree Harshitha Vallabhaneni, Sri Sravya Lalitha Chandrika Thungathurthi, Supraj Teeparthy, Winnie Long

First published in London, United Kingdom, 2025 by IntechOpen
IntechOpen is the global imprint of INTECHOPEN LIMITED, registered in England and Wales, registration number: 11086078, 167-169 Great Portland Street, London, W1W 5PF, United Kingdom

For EU product safety concerns: IN TECH d.o.o., Prolaz Marije Krucifikse Kozulić 3, 51000 Rijeka, Croatia, info@intechopen.com or visit our website at intechopen.com.

British Library Cataloguing-in-Publication Data
A catalogue record for this book is available from the British Library

Biliary Tract - Disease, Treatment, and Quality of Life
Edited by Qiang Yan
p. cm.
Print ISBN 978-0-85014-769-8
Online ISBN 978-0-85014-768-1
eBook (PDF) ISBN 978-0-85014-770-4

Meet the editor

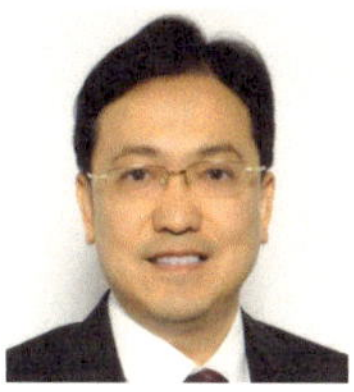

Qiang Yan, MD, FACS, is a Professor and Chief General Surgery Physician. He currently serves as Vice President of Huzhou Hospital, Zhejiang University School of Medicine, and Chairman of the National Clinical Key Specialty (Department of General Surgery). In 2019, he earned a certificate from the Surgical Leadership Program at Harvard Medical School in the United States. He became a Fellow of the American College of Surgeons in 2016 and was named a special member of the Japan-Germany Society for the Study of Liver Surgery in 2018.

Contents

Preface

Biliary tract diseases represent one of the most common clinical conditions encountered by hepatobiliary surgeons, encompassing congenital disorders, inflammatory diseases, and neoplastic conditions, which pose significant threats to human health. The challenges we face include diagnosing, treating, and improving the quality of life for patients. With advancements in science and technology, numerous innovative techniques and methods have emerged in recent years, leading to substantial improvements in therapeutic outcomes for these diseases. However, many aspects still require further enhancement. The authors of this book have invited renowned professors from around the world who have made outstanding contributions to the diagnosis and treatment of biliary tract diseases to provide in-depth discussions on these topics. We have also selected several high-quality papers with particular clinical significance and practical guidance, compiling them into this volume to offer readers valuable insights.

Qiang Yan
Zhejiang University,
Hangzhou, China

Chapter 1

Introductory Chapter: Biliary Tract-Disease, Treatment, and Quality of Life

Qiang Yan

1. Anatomy and physiological basis of biliary system

1.1 Composition of the biliary system

The biliary system consists of intrahepatic bile ducts, extrahepatic bile ducts, the gallbladder, and the sphincter of Oddi. The intrahepatic bile ducts originate from the capillary bile ducts and progressively converge into interlobular bile ducts, segmental bile ducts, and lobular bile ducts, ultimately forming the left and right hepatic ducts. The extrahepatic bile ducts consist of the common hepatic duct, cystic duct, and common bile duct. The common bile duct converges with the pancreatic duct to form the hepatopancreatic ampulla (Vater's ampulla), which terminates in the descending part of the duodenum. The pear-shaped gallbladder serves to store, concentrate, and evacuate bile. The cystic duct joins with the common hepatic duct to form the common bile duct. The sphincter of Oddi controls the release of bile and pancreatic juice through its contraction and relaxation.

1.2 Bile production and excretion

Bile is continuously secreted by hepatocytes, with a daily secretion volume of about 800 to 1200 ml. The main components of bile include bile salts, phospholipids, cholesterol, and bilirubin. Bile salts exert essential functions in fat digestion and absorption by emulsifying fats, increasing the contact area between fats and lipase, and promoting the absorption of fatty acids and glycerides. Bile secretion is regulated through neurohumoral pathways: Postprandial gastric acid, protein degradation products, and dietary fats stimulate the duodenal mucosal lining to release cholecystokinin (CCK) and secretin. CCK induces gallbladder contraction coupled with sphincter of Oddi relaxation, facilitating bile discharge into the duodenal lumen.

2. Common biliary diseases and their pathogenesis

2.1 Gallstones

2.1.1 Etiology and pathogenesis

The formation of gallstones is closely related to the imbalance of bile components, reduced gallbladder contraction function, and bacterial infection.

IntechOpen

Cholesterol/bilirubin supersaturation in bile initiates crystal nucleation, while delayed gallbladder evacuation predisposes to biliary stasis, compounded by bacterial-induced inflammatory cascades - all contributing to lithogenesis. Stone classification based on compositional predominance stratifies them into cholesterol stones (representing >80% of cases), pigment stones, and mixed variants.

2.1.2 Clinical manifestations

Most patients with gallstones are asymptomatic, termed "asymptomatic gallstones." When calculi obstruct the cystic duct or gallbladder neck, this can cause biliary colic, characterized by paroxysmal pain in the upper right abdomen, which may radiate to the right shoulder or back, often accompanied by nausea and vomiting. If secondary bacterial infection occurs, it can progress to acute cholecystitis, manifesting with systemic signs including pyrexia, rigors, and Murphy's sign (cessation of inspiration during gallbladder palpation).

2.2 Biliary calculi

2.2.1 Classification and etiology

Biliary calculi are stratified into intrahepatic and extrahepatic biliary stones. Extrahepatic biliary stones often result from gallstones migrating into the biliary tract, whereas intrahepatic biliary stones are associated with factors such as intrahepatic infection, bile stasis, and parasites (like *Clonorchis sinensis*). Intrahepatic lithiasis may induce progressive biliary strictures and hepatic parenchyma atrophy, increasing the difficulty of treatment.

2.2.2 Clinical manifestations

Biliary calculi, especially intrahepatic bile duct stones, are often asymptomatic. Extrahepatic bile duct stones and some intrahepatic bile duct stones may manifest with the Charcot triad: right upper quadrant pain, spiking fever with rigors, and obstructive jaundice. Ductal obstruction by calculi results in biliary stasis precipitating conjugated hyperbilirubinemia, while bacterial superinfection induces endotoxemia manifesting as systemic inflammatory response syndrome (SIRS). Progression to Reynold's pentad (Charcot's triad plus hypotension and altered mental status) signals acute obstructive suppurative cholangitis (AOSC), a life-threatening condition requiring emergent intervention. Early diagnosis and early relief of obstruction with unobstructed drainage are particularly emphasized in such diseases.

2.3 Cholecystitis

2.3.1 Acute cholecystitis

Acute cholecystitis predominantly arises from cystic duct obstruction by gallstones, with less frequent cases resulting from microbial infiltration of the gallbladder wall (commonly *Escherichia coli* and *Klebsiella* spp.). Pathologically, it demonstrates hyperemic, edematous, and exudative changes. Advanced cases may progress to gangrenous necrosis and carry the risk of transmural perforation.

2.3.2 Chronic cholecystitis

Chronic cholecystitis is often evolved from recurrent acute cholecystitis or chronic gallstone irritation of the gallbladder mucosa. Affected individuals may experience persistent right upper quadrant (RUQ) discomfort, postprandial epigastric fullness, and dyspeptic symptoms including belching. Notably, a significant patient subset remains clinically asymptomatic throughout disease progression.

2.4 Biliary tract tumors

2.4.1 Gallbladder cancer

Gallbladder carcinoma represents the most prevalent primary malignancy within the hepatobiliary system. Early-stage disease typically manifests with nonspecific clinical presentations, frequently masqueraded by coexisting cholelithiasis and chronic cholecystitis. In the advanced stage, jaundice, weight loss, and mass in the upper right abdomen may occur. Prognosis remains dismal, with 5-year survival rates <5% even with multimodal therapeutic approaches.

2.4.2 Cholangiocarcinoma

Cholangiocarcinoma originates from the biliary epithelium and is stratified into intrahepatic and extrahepatic subtypes. The main symptoms are progressive jaundice, refractory pruritus, and alcoholic stools. Established etiological factors encompass hepatolithiasis, primary sclerosing cholangitis (PSC), and congenital biliary malformations, with chronic inflammatory insults constituting the principal carcinogenic pathway.

3. Progress in diagnosis and treatment of biliary diseases

3.1 Diagnostic methods

3.1.1 Imaging examination

- Ultrasound examination: As we all know, it is the preferred method for biliary diseases. Ultrasound contrast examination can be carried out in combination with special contrast agents, which is of great help in distinguishing benign and malignant tumors.

- CT/MRI: can more accurately assess the extent of biliary cancer invasion, intrahepatic bile duct dilation, and metastasis. Magnetic resonance cholangiopancreatography (MRCP) is a non-invasive examination that can clearly show the anatomical structure of the biliary system.

- Endoscopic retrograde cholangiopancreatography (ERCP): both diagnostic and therapeutic functions, through the insertion of the duodenoscope into the bile duct, can directly observe the lesions of the bile duct and perform operations such as stone removal, biopsy, stent placement, etc. The advent of the second-generation SpyGlass digital system (DS) cholangioscope has provided a novel diagnostic approach for early-stage cholangiocarcinoma, biliary strictures, and bile duct stones [1].

- PET-CT/MRI: can further clarify the benign and malignant lesions of biliary tract tumors and the status of distant metastasis.
- The application of AI in imaging is becoming more and more extensive, which not only reduces clinical work pressure but also improves the accuracy of clinical diagnosis.

3.2 Laboratory examination

In addition to the common serum bilirubin, alkaline phosphatase (ALP), γ-glutamyl transferase (γ-GT), white blood cell count, C-reactive protein (CRP), carcinoembryonic antigen (CEA), carbohydrate antigen 19-9 (CA19-9) for the diagnosis of biliary diseases, the latest circulating tumor cells, peripheral blood RNA, cell gene sequencing also provide a lot of effective information.

3.3 Treatment methods

3.3.1 Surgical treatment

Conventional surgeries, including cholecystectomy, choledocholithotomy, and radical tumor resection, have evolved from open surgery to laparoscopic surgery and then to robotic surgery. Compared to traditional laparoscopy, robotic systems significantly enhance the precision of complex biliary tract tumor resections (such as hilar cholangiocarcinoma) and reduce risks of vascular and neural injury through three core technologies: 3D high-definition visualization, 7-degree-of-freedom robotic arms, and tremor filtration technology [2]. During this period, there was also a phase where extended resections were performed to achieve complete removal of the lesion. Today, we aim for surgeries that preserve maximum function (such as partial sphincter-preserving resection and reconstruction of the bile duct, and pancreaticoduodenectomy with duodenal preservation). Currently, there is a growing emphasis on minimally invasive approaches. The transumbilical single-incision laparoscopic cholecystectomy offers concealed postoperative scarring and reduced pain, effectively meeting the esthetic demands of young female patients [3].

3.3.2 Endoscopic treatment

ERCP can be used for gallbladder stone removal, biliary stricture dilation, and stent placement. For patients with cholangiocarcinoma who cannot undergo surgery, metal stents can be placed through ERCP to relieve jaundice and improve quality of life. The application of choledochoscopy in the management of bile duct stones significantly enhances stone clearance rates while reducing both patient discomfort and healthcare burden [4]. The novel stents offer innovative therapeutic strategies for disease management, including biodegradable polylactic acid (PLA) or polycaprolactone (PCL) stents, which degrade within 6–12 months and are utilized for benign biliary strictures to eliminate the need for secondary removal procedures [5], as well as radioactive seed-loaded covered metal stents incorporating iodine-125 particles, which simultaneously alleviate malignant obstructions and deliver localized radiotherapy to prolong stent patency and inhibit tumor progression [6].

3.3.3 Interventional treatment

Transperitoneal transhepatic biliary drainage (PTCD) is suitable for patients with obstructive jaundice who cannot tolerate surgery. The drainage tube is inserted through the puncture of intrahepatic bile duct to reduce jaundice symptoms. For intrahepatic bile duct stones, transperitoneal transhepatic cholangioscopy (PTCS) can be used.

3.3.4 Drug therapy

Antibiotics are used to control biliary tract infection; bile-promoting drugs can promote bile excretion and relieve symptoms; for patients with biliary tract tumors who cannot be operated, chemotherapy, targeted therapy, immune checkpoint inhibitors, and other treatments can be used.

4. The impact of biliary diseases on quality of life

4.1 Physiological function limitation

Patients with biliary diseases often suffer from abdominal pain, indigestion, jaundice, and other symptoms that affect eating and nutrient absorption, leading to weight loss and fatigue. Post-cholecystectomy, some patients develop steatorrhea, necessitating long-term dietary fat restriction. In advanced cholangiocarcinoma, due to liver failure, patients' ability to take care of themselves severely declines.

4.2 Psychological stress

Disease recurrence, surgical risks, and adverse prognostic outcomes in biliary malignancies predispose patients to psychiatric comorbidities, particularly anxiety and depressive disorders. Clinical observations consistently reveal multidimensional impairment of health-related quality of life (HRQOL) in biliary disease patients, paralleled by increased suicidality rates. This patient cohort demonstrates a disproportionate psychological burden, with one-third manifesting significantly greater distress levels than observed in other cancer populations [7].

4.3 Social dysfunction

Frequent medical treatment and long-term treatment lead to the decline of patients' working ability and the reduction of social activities. Pathophysiological manifestations such as jaundice and pruritus frequently engender impaired self-perception, creating psychosocial barriers that impede societal reintegration in susceptible individuals.

5. Strategies to improve quality of life

5.1 Diet management

Patients should follow the principles of low-fat and high-fiber diet, gradually increase fat intake, and avoid greasy and spicy food. Supplementing vitamin K (such as green leafy vegetables) can improve coagulation function; patients with intrahepatic lithiasis require specific dietary oxalate restriction, notably avoiding spinach and chocolate.

5.2 Psychological intervention

Psychoemotional distress in biliary disorders can be ameliorated through multimodal interventions including professional psychotherapy, structured family-system support, and peer-led support collectives. Cognitive behavioral therapy (CBT) can help patients adjust their perception of the disease and enhance coping ability.

5.3 Advances in treatment strategies

Modern medicine not only focuses on the diagnosis and treatment of diseases but also places increasing emphasis on improving patients' quality of life. Treatment strategies have evolved to become more precise and individualized, with progressively reduced adverse effects on normal physiological functions, enabling patients to recover more quickly.

5.4 Rehabilitation and follow-up

Patients after cholecystectomy should exercise appropriately to promote the recovery of gastrointestinal function; cholangiocarcinoma patients need regular review of tumor markers and imaging examinations to monitor the changes in the condition. During postoperative convalescence, digestive function can be improved through adjunctive Traditional Chinese Medicine (TCM) modalities (e.g., acupuncture therapy and herbal formulations).

6. Conclusion

Biliary system diseases constitute significant clinical challenges to global health, and their diagnosis and treatment require a comprehensive consideration of disease type and individual patient differences. With the development of minimally invasive techniques, endoscopic treatments, and molecularly targeted agents, treatment outcomes have significantly improved. However, improving patients' quality of life is equally important, necessitating intervention measures from physiological, psychological, and social dimensions. In the future, personalized therapy and precision medicine will bring more hope to patients with biliary diseases.

Author details

Qiang Yan
Zhejiang University, China

*Address all correspondence to: yanqiangdoc@hotmail.com

References

[1] Fugazza A, Gabbiadini R, Tringali A, et al. Digital single-operator cholangioscopy in diagnostic and therapeutic bilio-pancreatic diseases: A prospective, multicenter study. Digestive and Liver Disease. 2022;**54**:1243-1249. DOI: 10.1016/j.dld.2022.04.019

[2] Ratti F, Cipriani F, Ingallinella S, et al. Robotic approach for lymphadenectomy in biliary tumors: The missing ring between the benefits of laparoscopic and reproducibility of open approach? Annals of Surgery. 2023;**278**:e780-e788. DOI: 10.1097/SLA.0000000000005748

[3] Krollmann N, Hunger R, Paasch C, et al. Incidence of incisional hernias and cosmetic outcome after laparoscopic single-incision cholecystectomy: A long-term follow-up cohort study of 125 patients. Annals of Medicine and Surgery. 2024;**86**:50-55. DOI: 10.1097/MS9.0000000000001442

[4] Li G, Pang Q, Zhai H, et al. SpyGlass-guided laser lithotripsy versus laparoscopic common bile duct exploration for large common bile duct stones: A non-inferiority trial. Surgical Endoscopy. 2021;**35**:3723-3731. DOI: 10.1007/s00464-020-07862-4

[5] Chen A, Tey K, Verhage R, et al. Percutaneous biodegradable stent placement for treatment of benign biliary strictures: A systematic review. Journal of Vascular and Interventional Radiology. 2025;**36**:556-563. DOI: 10.1016/j.jvir.2024.12.595

[6] Huang YY, Xu XJ, Huang XZ, et al. A stent with radioactive seed strand insertion for inoperable malignant biliary obstruction: A meta-analysis. Brachytherapy. 2021;**20**:638-644. DOI: 10.1016/j.brachy.2021.01.010

[7] Graf J, Stengel A. Psychological burden and psycho-oncological interventions for patients with hepatobiliary cancers-a systematic review. Frontiers in Psychology. 2021;**12**:662777. DOI: 10.3389/fpsyg.2021.662777

Chapter 2

Alagille Syndrome in the Paediatric Population

Sabina Więcek

Abstract

Alagille syndrome (AGS) is a genetically determined condition affecting the liver and bile ducts, the cardiovascular system, the eyesight, the skeletal and/or the urinary systems. In most patients, the mutation of the JAG1 gene is responsible for the condition and less frequently *NOTCH gene*. The clinical picture is characterised by cholestasis, heart defects (most commonly pulmonary stenosis) and features of dysmorphia. The syndrome is diagnosed based on the symptoms and results of specialist tests and confirmed by the result of genetic tests JAG1 (jagged canonical notch ligant1) or NOTCH (neurogenic locus notch homolog protein). mutation. If untreated, Alagille syndrome leads to cirrhosis and liver failure. The new treatment options, which have become available in the form of sodium-dependent bile acid transporter inhibitors, may improve the prognosis as well as the patient's quality of life, and may prevent the need for liver transplant in this group of patients.

Keywords: Alagille syndrome, children, symptoms, diagnostic procedure, therapeutic procedure

1. Introduction

Alagille syndrome (AGS) is a congenital, genetically determined multisystemic disease that presents with bile duct paucity, congenital heart defects, as well as defects of the spine, the eyesight, kidneys and features of dysmorphia. It was first described by Dr. Daniel Alagille in 1962 (*Congenital absence of the intrahepatic bile ducts*) [1–8].

2. Aetiology and aetiopathogenesis

Alagille syndrome is caused by mutations (or deletions) within two main genes, namely JAG1 (responsible for around 90–95% of cases)—coding for the JAGGED1 protein—a ligand for the NOTCH receptors, and less frequently NOTCH2—coding for one of the NOTCH receptors (~2.5%). Ninety-five per cent of patients show heterozygous expression of the JAG1 gene—15% are missense mutations (mainly cysteine), and in 85% of cases it involves shortening of the protein chain. As many as 2.5% of patients show the heterozygous variant of the NOTCH2 gene—68% of missense mutations, and in 32% of cases it involves shortening of the protein chain. Disruption in the JAG1/NOTCH signalling pathway, which is necessary for the process of cellular differentiation during embryogenesis, contributes to the abnormal development of many tissues and organs, including the intrahepatic bile ducts. The JAG1 gene mutation (Jagged 1 proteins) involves transmembrane protein combined with epidermal growth factor (EGF) [9].

Alagille syndrome is inherited in an autosomal dominant pattern. In about 60% of cases, *de novo* mutations are reported. So far, no correlation between the type of mutation and the clinical picture (genotype → phenotype) has been observed. The clinical picture may vary, even within one family [10–17].

3. Epidemiology

The occurrence of Alagille syndrome is estimated at 1/70,000 live births but it appears to be greater (1/30,000), with the former number being the result of underdiagnosis [7, 8, 11, 17–20].

4. Clinical manifestations

The systemic lesions most commonly include the liver and the bile ducts, the cardiovascular system, the eyesight, the skeletal system and features of facial dysmorphia. The clinical picture of Alagille syndrome is shown in **Table 1**.

Other symptoms of Alagille syndrome include: growth failure, laryngological and/or endocrine complications.

To confirm the diagnosis of Alagille syndrome, it is necessary to confirm three main features or two in patients with a family history of the condition [1, 5, 7, 10, 11, 13, 15, 16, 21].

4.1 Cholestasis

Cholestasis usually occurs in the first weeks of life. Acholic stools and increased activity of gamma-glutamyl transpeptidase (GGTP) are observed in some patients, so biliary atresia should always form part of the differential diagnosis. In clinically uncertain situations, histopathological examination must be performed. Biliary paucity is observed in children with Alagille syndrome, which affects the peripheral parts of the liver in particular (lesions in the central part are relatively less advanced) [6, 7, 16, 17, 21–23]. Hepatic regenerative nodules are observed in patients with Alagille syndrome, but they are thought to be a functional adaptation to vascular changes rather than a neoplastic process. The nodules are typically centrally located and normal hepatic vasculature coursing through the lesions is noted radiologically. Microscopically, they are characterised by circumscribed hepatic lesions with preserved architecture, lesser degrees of fibrosis and relative preservation of interlobular bile ducts compared to the background cirrhotic liver [22–24]. These nodules should be distinguished from hepatocellular carcinoma (HCC) and adenoma because there is a decreased risk of hepatocellular carcinoma (HCC) in patients with Alagille syndrome [22, 24, 25]. Other histological findings observed in the liver biopsies in patients with Alagille syndrome include hepatocanalicular bilirubinostasis with

System	Symptoms/clinical picture
1. Liver and bile ducts (75–100%)	Bile duct paucity Cholestasis Pruritus
2. Cardiovascular system (85–98%)	Peripheral pulmonary artery stenosis—most frequent Pulmonary stenosis Complex heart defects—e.g., tetralogy of Fallot (TOF) Atrial septal defect (ASD) Ventricular septal defect (VSD) Lesions in the peripheral vessels, e.g., central nervous system (CNS)
3. Skeletal system (33–87%)	Butterfly vertebrae Hemivertebrae Fusion of adjacent vertebra Spina bifida occulta Short distal phalanges of the fingers Insufficient growth
4. Ocular (56–88%)	Posterior embryotoxon—abnormality of the posterior chamber Optic disc drusen Defects of the iris Pigmentary retinopathy Angulated retinal vessels
5. Facial dysmorphia (70–98%)	Broad forehead Deep-set eyes Bulbous tipped nose Upslanting palpebral fissures Prominent ears Pointed chin Underdeveloped earlobes (rarely) Cleft palate (rarely)
6. Urinary system (17–73%)	Kidney dysplasia Posterior urethral valve Renal tubular acidosis Kidney cysts
7. Vascular system (4–38%)	30% abnormalities in the internal carotid artery 20% cerebral aneurysms Aneurysm of intra-abdominal vessels Increases the risk of stroke Moya-moya disease Intracranial bleeding

Table 1.
Clinical manifestations of Alagille syndrome.

resetting, patchy giant cell transformation, haemopoiesis and variable portal inflammation. Malnutrition, deficiency in fat-soluble vitamins, blood-clotting disorders and osteopenia are observed as a result of cholestasis. As the condition progresses, in most children a persistent skin itch develops together with cirrhosis and portal hypertension (relatively late). The development of portal hypertension is proportional to the levels of bilirubin (with concentration levels of bilirubin in blood serum at 5–10 mg/dL—it is 4 times greater, >10 mg/dL 8× greater risk) [21–26].

Increased skin itch occurs in a large proportion of patients, which contributes to the following:

a. Problems falling asleep and sleeping

b. Impaired concentration—poor scholastic

c. Lower mood and self-esteem

d. Discomfort

e. Lichenification of skin and secondary infections

The aetiopathogenesis of this increased skin itch is not fully understood; however, high concentration levels of bile acids (especially hydrophobic, unconjugated), lysophosphatidic acid (LPA), lysophosphatidylcholine (LPC), steroids (derivatives of pregnanediol) and elevated levels of bilirubin undoubtedly play a role [13, 18, 21, 25–27].

Splenomegaly is observed in 30–70% of patients, usually occurring secondary to portal hypertension.

4.2 Cardiovascular system

Most common abnormalities concern the cardiovascular system of the right-hand side and include pulmonary artery hypoplasia (PAH), tetralogy of Fallot (TOF) and pulmonary stenosis. Pulmonary stenosis is the most common complication and accounts for around 67% of heart defects. Heart defects are very often detected as early as during prenatal testing. No correlation between the type of JAG1 gene mutation and the type of anomaly within the cardiovascular system has been shown. Pulmonary arteries show features of the narrowing of the lumen of arteries as a result of the thickening of the middle section, an increased number of elastic fibres and internal membrane overgrowth caused by proliferating smooth muscle cells. Vascular lesions often occur in this group of patients (in around 10%) and include strictures, aneurysms within the central nervous system, the jugular veins, the aorta and renal arteries. The presence of vascular lesions in the group of patients with Alagille syndrome significantly deteriorates their prognosis and increases the mortality rate. It is worth noting that that the presence of vascular lesions in Alagille syndrome highlights the significance of the *Jagged1* gene and NOTCH in the formation of vessels. Systemic and cerebrovascular vasculopathy undoubtedly plays a role [28–32].

Unfortunately, it has been proved that the intra- and postoperative course in patients with a heart defect in Alagille syndrome is worse than in patients without AGS. Liver transplant can be performed before or after reducing the stricture in the pulmonary artery depending on the pressure in the right ventricle and the heart's ability to sustain increased output [28–32].

4.3 Kidneys and the urinary and reproductive system

NOTCH2 is expressed in renal tubular and glomerular epithelia, while JAGGED1 is expressed over the endothelium of glomeruli collecting tubules in a fully formed nephron. It has been proved that mice, which are homozygous carriers of the NOTCH2 gene, have defects of the glomerular blood vessels, podocytes and the proximal ureters. The impact of the NOTCH gene mutation on acute and chronic kidney damage has also been confirmed. The most common renal complications in patients with Alagille syndrome are:

a. CAKUT—congenital anomalies of kidney and urinary tract—renal agenesis, hypoplasia, dysplasia, renal cysts, hydronephrosis and ureteropelvic junction obstruction

b. Proteinuria

c. Renovascular hypertension

d. Proximal renal tubular defect (RTA)

e. Renal tubular acidosis

Kidney biopsy is rarely performed. The histopathological examination most often reveals glomerular mesangiolipidosis-like lesions. They correlate with intensified cholestasis and the concentration level of cholesterol and triglycerides in the blood serum. Sometimes the following are observed: glomerular basement membrane lipidosis, biliary nephropathy and/or focal glomerulosclerosis and small kidney cysts. Renal tubular acidosis is characteristic for Alagille syndrome and it also affects the absorption of calcium and contributes to abnormalities in bone mineralisation, the process of growth and weight gain [18, 31, 33, 34].

The observed hypertension may be of a vascular nature (renal vasculopathy). Unfortunately, no preventative methods are available. Blood pressure has to be checked on a regular basis in patients with Alagille syndrome. Parameters of kidney function, such as creatinine, urea, electrolytes in the blood serum, gas analysis, general urinalysis, urine protein/albumin excretion and kidney ultrasound (a minimum of once a year), also have to be checked regularly. Periodically, it is also important to perform Doppler ultrasound and angioCT or angioMRI in questionable cases. If any abnormalities are noticed, the patient should be referred to a nephrologist. The use of ACEI/ARB (angiotensin converting enzyme inhibitors/angiotensin II receptor antagonists) should be cautious. It has to be highlighted that patients with Alagille syndrome and liver failure have a high risk of developing kidney failure as a result of the hepatorenal syndrome [28, 33, 34].

4.4 Central nervous system

4.4.1 Vascular lesions

NOTCH plays an important role in angiogenesis, as it is expressed by vascular endothelium during embryogenesis. This could explain the predisposition to develop vascular abnormalities. According to Kamath, over 30% of patients with Alagille syndrome have abnormalities within the central nervous system, including changes in the vessels (over 30% involve abnormalities in the internal carotid artery and 20% cerebral aneurysms). Abnormalities within the vertebral arteries are reported in around 10%. In 16% of patients, increase in the risk of stroke is observed, but it is not a common feature in children under 16 years of age. Cerebral aneurysms are slightly higher in males. CT/MRI scans should be performed in patients with Alagille syndrome in the case of head trauma or the occurrence of new abnormal neurological symptoms. Additionally, it is recommended to perform angioCT before liver transplantation. Central nervous system bleeding is observed in around 15% of patients. It is intracranial bleeding that is responsible for 25–50% of deaths of patients with AGS. Ischaemic strokes are also more frequently observed in this group of patients. Some authors postulate that an MRI of the CNS should be done in every patient with AGS over the age of 8 years when a general anaesthetic is no longer necessary. The scan should be repeated every 5 years [8, 10, 19, 26, 28–31].

4.4.2 Psychomotor development

Impairment of the psychomotor activity in children with AGS is described in the subject literature. The mean intelligence quotient (IQ) in patients with Alagille syndrome is lower, and some of them require special education. Its course and frequency of occurrence are comparable with those of the group of patients with biliary atresia. Patients with Alagille syndrome are also known to have higher incidence of attention deficit hyperkinetic disorder, depression, anxiety and eating disorders. The following factors may have an impact: frequent hospitalisations, medical interventions, increased skin itch and in older patients low self-esteem (e.g., caused by the features of dysmorphia) and lower quality of life [35–38].

4.4.3 Malformations of the cranium and the facial skeleton

The loss of the Jagged1 protein in the cranial sutures may cause craniosynostosis and progressing plagiocephaly. The expression of *NOTCH* in the human jaw cartilage is high. Idiopathic intracranial hypertension has also been reported in Alagille syndrome. Pathogenesis is still not defined but it can be related to craniosynostosis. As well, as it may influence cerebrospinal fluid (CSF) production due to its involvement in angiogenesis [7, 8, 10, 16, 37].

4.4.4 The normal functioning of the Jagged1-Notch gene has been proved to be crucial for the development of the inner ear and thus hearing

Defects of the stirrup and the cochlea of the inner ear, leading to impaired hearing, are observed in Alagille syndrome [5, 7, 8, 10, 26, 31].

4.4.5 Ophthalmologic abnormalities

Ophthalmologic abnormalities mainly concern the front section of the eye, with posterior embryotoxon (PE) affecting over 80% of patients with AGS. Posterior embryotoxon (PE) is a corneal abnormality that is visible with slit-lamp biomicroscopy as a thin grey-white, arcuate ridge on the inner surface of the cornea, adjacent to the limbus. It is an anteriorly displaced Schwalbe's line, the junction of Descemet's membrane and the uveal trabecular meshwork. Histologically, it consists of a central collagen core surrounded by a thin layer of Descemet's membrane and is separated from the anterior chamber by a layer of endothelium. Abnormalities concerning the optic nerve or the retina (its peripheral part) occur relatively rarely. The first symptoms involve difficulty seeing in the dark and impaired peripheral vision. There have been reports of lens subluxation in patients with Alagille syndrome [7, 8, 16, 39, 40].

5. Other abnormalities

a. *Bone abnormalities*—structural abnormalities, lower bone mass, fractures. The *NOTCH* gene regulates the osteoblastic and the osteoclastic differentiation, and the bone remodelling in the early stages of development. Abnormalities within the skeletal system are summarised in **Table 2** [5, 31, 41].

b. *Insufficient growth and body weight*—impaired growth is observed in 50–87% of cases. In most patients, insufficient body weight and/or growth is observed from the foetal stage of development. Two thirds of children are born with lower than expected body weight and height. The aetiopathogenesis of growth insufficiency in patients with Alagille syndrome is very complex. Reduced muscle and fat mass is observed. The concentration levels of the growth hormone and the growth hormone-binding protein are elevated in patients with Alagille syndrome; however, the number of growth hormone receptors and insulin-like growth factor 1 (IGF-1) receptors is reduced. Additional factors involve malabsorption and digestive disorders (cholestasis, pancreatic insufficiency and food neophobia), increased need for (circulatory insufficiency, ESLD—end-stage liver disease) and insufficient supply of nutrients and calories (lack of appetite, increased skin itch). The occurrence of insufficient body weight and height in children with Alagille syndrome is also affected by anomalies in the circulatory system, the kidneys, CNS and cholestasis [42, 43].

Skeletal abnormalities	Characteristic
Butterfly vertebrae	39–87% of patients Consequence of early stage developmental defects Characterised by the presence of the central sagittal cleft in the vertebral body, caused by failed fusion of lateral chondrification centres during spinal embryogenesis. Most often concerns the thoracic and lumbar spine Most frequently asymptomatic Multiple even in 40–48%
Other abnormalities of the vertebrae	Hemivertebrae, fusion of adjacent vertebrae (may be related to spinal deformation) Narrowing of disc space in the lumbar spine
Abnormal bone density	Reduced ability of bone regeneration Impaired osteoblastic and osteoclastic differentiation
Proneness to fractures	Impaired osteoblastic and osteoclastic differentiation Abnormalities in bone regeneration / remodelling Very frequent fractures without a cause or following a minor incident Most frequent in children below the age of 13
Craniofacial dysmorphism	Deep-set eyes Broad forehead Mild hypertelorism Small cheeks Sometimes cleft lip and palate Significant dysmorphic features require plastic surgery.
Scoliosis	
Abnormal fusions between adjacent ribs and forearm bones	
Shortening of the distal phalanges and of the ulna	

Table 2.
Abnormalities of the skeletal system in Alagille syndrome.

Special growth and body weight centile charts have been developed for patients with Alagille syndrome and should be used when assessing this group of paediatric patients. Meagre height significantly reduces the quality of life. It has been proved that insufficient body height and weight correlates with intensified cholestasis. However, when comparing patients with biliary atresia and Alagille syndrome with those with AGS, malnutrition, insufficient height (the average values are higher) and ascites are less frequently observed. In his study, Rovner confirmed a higher occurrence of deficiency body height and mass in patients with Alagille syndrome. He proved greater faecal fat losses in over 90% of patients, lower calorie intake in the diet (in particular in those with heart defects) and more frequent fat-soluble vitamin deficiency [42, 43]. Exocrine pancreatic insufficiency, which can be confirmed by measuring the amount of fat and elastase in faeces, is confirmed in around 40% of patients. Supplementing the diet with pancreatic enzyme proves useful in some patients. So far, no correlations between insufficient height and anomalies in the skeletal system have been shown. Therapy with IGF-1 has been attempted on this group of patients but has been unsuccessful [41–43].

c. *Anomalies within the oral cavity* involve a change in the number of teeth (in particular of canines), abnormal milk/permanent tooth eruption and position, changes in the shape and size of the teeth, enamel hypomineralisation, additional cusps [44].

d. *Endocrine disorders*. Abnormal functioning of the hypothalamic-pituitary-gonadal axis and secondary disorders of the metabolism of oestrogens are observed in this group of patients. Hypogonadism was first described by Alagille. Secondary period abnormalities and even lack of menstruation are observed in women [1, 2, 18, 27]. NOTCH signalling in thyrocytes is crucial for the normal functioning of thyroid in adults.

e. *Disorders of the lipid metabolism*. Elevated levels of total cholesterol (sometimes as high as 500 mg%) and the low-density lipoprotein (LDL) fraction and triglycerides (TGs) in the blood serum are observed in patients with Alagille syndrome. Additionally, the concentration levels of phospholipids and lipoprotein X are elevated. The pathomechanism of hypercholesterolaemia involves the abnormal binding of the bile with the Farnesoid X receptor (FXR), which hinders the production of bile acids and leads to the inability to excrete cholesterol. Cholesterol and phospholipids migrate to the bloodstream where they bind with albumins. Because of its size, lipoprotein X cannot penetrate the vessel wall like very low-density lipoprotein-cholesterol (VLDL-C) and so it continues to circulate in the bloodstream. Also, lipoprotein X cannot reach the liver via the LDL/ApoB (apolipoprotein B) receptor, so it accumulates in the blood and causes hypercholesterolaemia. Additionally, cholestasis disrupts the lipid metabolism by inducing 3-hydroxy-3-methyl-glutaryl-coenzyme A reductase (HMG-CoA reductase), increasing the expression of the LDL receptor and reducing the expression of liver cytochrome P-450 7A1 (CYP7A1) (reducing the conversion of cholesterol to bile acids). It must be remembered that elevated concentration levels of lipoprotein X/triglycerides cause pseudohyponatraemia in the blood serum. The pharmacological treatment with statins, PCXK9 antagonists or cholestyramine of this form of hypercholesterolaemia is ineffective. There are ongoing studies on the use of low doses of atorvastatin, which reduce the LDL-cholesterol by inhibiting the HMG-CoA reductase and improving the production and secretion of bile acids in this group of patients. Xanthomas occur in 20–42% of patients with Alagille syndrome. They most often develop at the age of 20–48 months in patients with severe jaundice. The presence of xanthomas and accompanying high concentration of cholesterol (about 500 mg%) is an adverse prognostic factor. Their intensity reduces as the liver function improves, with age and following the procedure of partial external biliary drainage or liver transplant [5, 17, 18, 20, 31, 45].

So far, the impact of hypercholesterolaemia on atherosclerotic lesions in patients with Alagille syndrome has not been proved. Lipoprotein X does not have atherogenic properties. However, Nagasaka et al. proved that through its antioxidant action, it has protective properties and additionally, it increases the concentration levels of the high-density lipoprotein-cholesterol (HDL-C) [45].

The role of immune disorders (cluster of differentiation 46 (CD46)) in patients with Alagille syndrome has been stressed. Twenty-five per cent of patients have recurrent infections of the respiratory tract. However, the incidence of postliver transplantation infections is similar to that of patients suffering from other aetiologies leading to advanced liver disease. The defective Jagged gene would also increase T helper 2 (TH2) cells, predisposing patients to asthma, food allergy and atopic dermatitis [29, 33, 46, 47].

During the ESPGHAN 2024 congress, the participants discussed the importance of the NOTCH gene mutation, including new variants for the aetiopathogenesis of Alagille syndrome, the natural history of liver lesions, extrahepatic manifestations and the latest treatment options with ileal bile acid transporter (IBAT) inhibitors. A significant amount of new information about the Alagille syndrome was offered by the multi-centre Global Alagille Alliance (GALA) study. The data were shared by Binita Kamath. Out of 931 patients with Alagille syndrome, only 34 carried the NOTCH2 mutation and this group was predominantly male. Patients who carried the NOTCH2 mutation during infancy in over 90% of cases presented with cholestasis in the neonatal period and in 60% of cases with biliary paucity. When the phenotype of the patients with NOTCH2 and JAGGED was compared, less frequent occurrence of the characteristic phenotype (56.3 vs. 90.1%) was concluded, as well as of heart defects (60.7 vs. 92.1%) and butterfly vertebrae (3.3 vs. 44.1%). Posterior embryotoxon was also less frequently diagnosed (18.5 vs. 53.1%) [19, 48].

6. Diagnostics

A thorough interview involving the medical history and a physical examination (features of dysmorphia, heart murmurs, cholestasis) plays a major role in the diagnostic process, as they may provide directions towards the correct diagnosis.

The results of laboratory tests revealed elevated parameters of cholestasis (elevated levels of bilirubin with dominant direct bilirubin and of bile acids and increased activity of gamma-glutamyl transpeptidase and alkaline phosphatase (ALP) in blood serum) as well as elevated parameters of liver damage (increased activity of aminotransferases). Hypercholesterolaemia is diagnosed in some patients. Blood-clotting disorders in the form of increased prothrombin time (INR) are quite frequently observed in young patients in particular, and require intravenous (iv) administration of vitamin K [7, 8, 10, 13, 20, 31, 46, 47].

Liver biopsy is not usually needed and is performed in clinically doubtful situations when it is impossible to come to a conclusive diagnosis. Histopathological examination of Alagille syndrome reveals biliary paucity and a lowered ratio of the number of interlobular bile ducts in relation to portal triads in and around 30% of biopsy specimens collected from infants. In rare cases, it may suggest biliary atresia (stalling of the bile flow, giant cell hepatitis, proliferation of the bile ducts) [20, 21, 46]. Unfortunately, sometimes as a result of a wrong diagnosis, patients with Alagille syndrome undergo the procedure of Kasai portoenterostomy.

Molecular testing proves very useful and contributes to a conclusive diagnosis, in particular in clinically doubtful situations [8, 14, 15, 17, 18]. Above 700 pathogenic variants in JAG1 and above 20 pathogenic variants in NOTCH2 have been reported in individuals with clinical features of Alagille syndrome.

7. Differential diagnostics

Differential diagnostics should always include cholestatic disorders with elevated activity of GGTP, especially biliary atresia and alpha 1-antitrypsin deficiency. The clinical picture and results of laboratory tests in both cases may be very similar.

8. Treatment

8.1 Management of pruritus

a. Bile secretion-promoting drugs—UDCA-ursodeoxycholic acid

b. Bile acid-binding drugs—cholestyramine

c. Antibiotics—rifampicin

d. Inhibitor of sodium-dependent bile acid transporter (ileal bile acid transporter). Ileal bile acid transporter (IBAT) reabsorbs about 95% of the synthesised bile acids when secreted into the small intestine. Maralixibat (Livmarli) and odevixibat (Bylvay) are IBAT blockers, and both are important treatment options for Alagille syndrome, the use of which can lead to significant reductions in the severity of pruritus. The most common adverse events reported across the trials included in this study were gastrointestinal (mainly diarrhoea and/or abdominal pain), which was likely due to the mechanism of action of IBAT blockers [48–51].

Maralixibat is approved by the Food and Drug Administration (FDA) and European Medicines Agency (EMA) for the treatment of children with Alagille syndrome below the age of 2 months. The recommended dose is 380 μg/kg of body weight 1 time/day. Maralixibat acts locally in the small intestine reducing the reuptake of bile acids from the distal ileum to liver portal circulation. Therefore, it lowers the concentration levels of bile acids in the blood and the liver, leading to the alleviation of the symptoms of pruritus [26, 47–51].

In clinical studies currently being conducted on children, there are other inhibitors of sodium-dependent bile acid transporters: odevixibat. Odevixibat is a small-molecule inhibitor of the ileal bile acid transporter being developed for the treatment of various cholestatic diseases, including Progressive Familial Intrahepatic Cholestasis (PFIC) and Alagille syndrome [51, 52].

During the ESPGHAN conference 2024, Terner-Rosenthal showed the data concerning the impact of the use of maralixibat on the need to use other anti-pruritus drugs in patients with Alagille syndrome. Because of the intensity of pruritus and its significant impact on the quality of life in this group of patients, the following drugs are often used: ursodeoxycholic acid, rifampicin and antihistamines. The presented data concerned 116 patients treated with maralixibat for at least a year as part of the ICONIC (Conservative versus Conventional oxygenation targets in intensive care patients) double-blind study. Following the reduction in the intensity of pruritus in 35% of patients, one drug was stopped, in 19%—two drugs and in 6%—three drugs [48, 49, 53]. Sturm showed the data from the 3rd stage of a double-blind, randomised ASSERT (The Asymptomatic Atrial Fibrillation and Stroke Evaluation in Pacemaker Patients and the Atrial Fibrillation Reduction Atrial Pacing Trial) and open-label ASSERT-EXT trial that included patients with genetically confirmed Alagille syndrome (with JAG1 or NOTCH2 mutation). It involved patients treated with odevixibat for 48 weeks [54]. Similar to previous reports, a statistically significant reduction in the concentration of bile acids in the serum and in the intensity of pruritus as well as improved quality of

Drug	Dosage	Adverse reactions
Choleretics Ursodeoxycholic acid UDCA- hepatoprotective, cholangioprotective	10–20 mg/kg of body weight	Diarrhoea, abdominal pain
Bile acid sequestrants Cholestyramine Nonabsorbable anion exchange resin: binds with bile acids	240 mg/kg/24 h (max 8 g/24 h)	Constipation, abdominal pain, diarrhoea, metabolic acidosis, absorption disorders
Antibiotics—Rifampicin cytochrome P-450 induction 6 α hydroxylation of bile acids	10 mg/kg/24 h (max 600 mg/24 h)	Reddish discolouration of body fluids Allergic reactions Increased activity of aminotransferases CAUTIOUS approach is needed due to its interactions with other drugs
Antihistamines Hydroxyzine Diphenhydramine	2 mg/kg/24 h 5 mg/kg/24 h	Drowsiness Difficulty concentrating
Opioid antagonists Naltrexone	0.25–0.5 mg/kg (max 50 mg)	Opioid withdrawal symptoms
Selective serotonin reuptake inhibitors (SSRIs) Sertraline	1–4 mg/kg/24 h (max 200 mg/24 h)	Behavioural changes Skin lesions Vomiting Hypertension
Inhibitor of sodium-dependent bile acid transporter E.g., Maralixibat Odevixibat	380 μg/kg/24 h	Temporary diarrhoea, abdominal pain

Table 3.
Pharmacological treatment of pruritus.

life/sleep was observed. Diarrhoea was the most common adverse reaction to the treatment; however, it subsided once the medication was withdrawn [50–57]. IBAT receptors participate in the absorption of the majority of bile acids in the ileum. Some of the conjugated bile acids, which are not absorbed in the small intestine, may be converted by the bacteria in the large intestine to unconjugated and secondary bile acids. These acids are absorbed without the participation of IBAT. The concentration levels of bile acids in the serum of the patients before the inclusion of odevixibat and after 24 weeks of treatment were analysed. Before the treatment, the concentration levels of primary unconjugated bile acids—the cholic acid (CA) and the chenodeoxycholic acid (CDCA) in the serum were low, probably because of the small amount of bile acids reaching the large intestine. After the treatment, a significant increase in the concentration of CA and CDCA in the serum was observed. Reduction in the total concentration levels of bile acids in the serum with the concurrent increase in the concentration levels of CA and CDCA may indicate the presence of bile acids in the large intestine and their deconjugation following the treatment with odevixibat [58].

Pharmacological treatment in Alagille syndrome is shown in **Table 3**.

Dietary treatment (prevention of malnutrition). A high-calorie diet is recommended (commercially available high-calorie food mixes), enriched with medium-chain triglycerides (MCT)-fat containing foods (C6-C10) or direct administration of MCT fats. Supplementation with calcium and pancreatic enzymes may sometimes be beneficial. In some patients, it may be necessary to administer food via a nasogastric feeding tube or percutaneous endoscopic gastrostomy (PEG). The feeding may be intensified by increasing the number of meals, their volume or introduction of night feeding with the use of a peristaltic pump. The possibility of portal hypertension and ruptured oesophageal/gastric varices, and haemorrhage has to be considered before the insertion of the tube [13, 18, 20, 33].

Supplementation with fat-soluble vitamins, ADEK (Vitamins A, D, E and K), including the oral/intravenous administration of vitamin K *to manage clotting disorders.*

Treatment of portal hypertension—endoscopic variceal banding.

8.2 Surgical procedures

1. Partial external biliary diversion (PEBD). The procedure of partial external biliary diversion/partial internal biliary diversion (PEBD/PIBD) is an alternative for liver transplant in patients with drug-resistant pruritus and those with intensified xanthomas but without cirrhosis and portal hypertension. Its efficiency is linked to a reduced amount of bile salts as a result of their increased loss due to PEBD, reduced renal excretion of bile salts and an increase in synthesis.

2. Liver transplant. Liver transplant is necessary in 20–50% of patients with Alagille syndrome. It accounts for around 5% of all liver transplants in children.

3. The most frequent indications for liver transplants (LTs) are:

    a. Acute liver failure-cirrhosis/portal hypertension—approx. 75%

    b. Complications in cholestasis: chronic intense pruritus (7%), insufficient growth (12%), osteopenia and pathological fractures (2%), drug-resistant blood-clotting disorders, multiple xanthomas or hepatocellular carcinoma [21, 26, 46, 59–61].

It is to be noted that the disease does not recur in the graft. Celiac artery stenosis and a hypoplastic hepatic artery are commonly noted in Alagille syndrome and hence an extra-anatomical arterial inflow may be required. Due to inherent renal involvement as a part of genetic syndrome, patients postliver transplantation have a higher risk of developing calcineurin inhibitor-induced nephrotoxicity.

The functioning of the kidneys and the cardiovascular system, as well as the perioperative care and immunosuppressive therapy, plays a crucial role. Currently, the 5-year survival rate following liver transplant in children with Alagille syndrome is 92%, the 10-year—91.2% and 18-year—88.1%. Comorbid heart defects and vascular lesions undoubtedly have an impact (over 33% of deaths). Right ventricular ischaemic lesions and a drop in the systemic pressure resulting from right ventricular hypertrophy are observed in children with AGS after the procedure [16, 17, 60–64].

It has been shown that accidentally done Kasai portoenterostomy for patients with Alagille syndrome-misdiagnosed biliary atresia leads to poor outcomes. A previous analysis had shown higher mortality (31 vs. 2.8%) and higher rate of liver transplantation (47.6 vs. 13.9%).

Perhaps in the future, the number of patients requiring a liver transplant will be decreasing as a result of the introduction of treatment with inhibitors of sodium-dependent bile acid transporters, such as maralixibat and odevixibat [47–51].

9. Pregnancy

Pregnancy can pose significant risk to expectant females with Alagille syndrome and the foetus. Physiological increase in cardiac output due to splanchnic and portal compression by the growing uterus may worsen portal hypertension in pregnancy, which can be linked to increase in variceal bleeding during pregnancy, higher rates of prematurity and spontaneous early abortion [8]. Similarly, haemodynamic changes associated with pregnancy may cause cardiac function to deteriorate in patients with pulmonary hypertension. Delivery via caesarean section or assisted vaginal delivery (forceps or vacuum) has been suggested as the delivery route in patients with portal hypertension, severe cardiac disease or intracranial vasculopathy [8]. Alagille syndrome in woman can lead to consequences, such as vitamin K deficiency, bleeding in the newborn, maxillary hypoplasia, foetal hypocalcaemia, intrauterine growth restriction (IUGR) and hypoproteinaemia.

10. Prognosis and natural course

Prognostic factors in patients with Alagille syndrome involve the complexity of the cardiovascular defects and the intensity of cholestasis. Kidney diseases and intracranial vascular lesions also play an important role. They are the most frequent causes of death in patients with Alagille syndrome. The overall 20-year survival rate is 62–88%. Hepatocarcinoma is more often seen in patients with Alagille syndrome than in the general population. The Notch pathway plays a major role in hepatic cellular differentiation, which in the setting of progressive fibrosis, may result in HCC tumourigenesis and progression. By 2020, 35 such cases were described, and only in half of them the cancer had a cirrhotic background. In one fourth of patients, the level of alpha fetoprotein (AFP) was normal. This is why patients with AGS require

AFP screening and regular liver scans. There is some uncertainty as to the frequency of such tests—the recommendation is every 6 months.

Patients with Alagille syndrome have a significantly lower quality of life, including the psychosocial aspect of life and poor physical activity. Depressive and anxiety episodes, self-harming and educational problems are more frequently observed compared to the general population [25, 30, 33, 37, 55, 62–64].

Alagille syndrome is a fascinating disease with multiple manifestations involving major organ systems spanning from infancy to adulthood.

To conclude, the prognosis of patients with Alagille syndrome is uncertain and currently there are no laboratory or genetic prognostic factors for this group of patients. Patients with Alagille syndrome require multispecialist care involving a gastroenterologist, a cardiologist, an eye specialist, a nephrologist, and an orthopaedic specialist, a dietician and other specialists [38, 46, 62–64].

Author details

Sabina Więcek
Faculty of Health Sciences, Department of Paediatrics, Medical University of Silesia, Upper-Silesian Child Health Centre, Katowice, Poland

*Address all correspondence to: sabinawk@wp.pl

References

[1] Alagille D. Alagille syndrome today. Clinical and Investigative Medicine. 1996;**19**(5):325-330

[2] Alagille D, Le Tan V. Congenital absence of the intrahepatic bile ducts. Revue Médico-Chirurgicale des Maladies du Foie. 1962;**37**:57-70

[3] Alagille D, Odievre M, Gautier M, et al. Hepatic ductular hypoplasia associated with characteristic facies, vertebral malformations, retarded physical, mental, and sexual development, and cardiac murmur. The Journal of Pediatrics. 1975;**86**(1):63-71

[4] Alagille D, Estrada A, Hadchouel M, et al. Syndromic paucity of interlobular bile ducts (Alagille syndrome or arteriohepatic dysplasia) review of 80 cases. The Journal of Pediatrics. 1987;**110**(2):195-200

[5] Jesina D. Alagille syndrome: An overview. Neonatal Network. 2017;**1;36**(6):343-347. DOI: 10.1891/0730-0832.36.6.343

[6] Ayoub M, Kamath B. Alagille syndrome: Current understanding of pathogenesis, and challenges in diagnosis and management. Clinics in Liver Disease. 2022;**26**(3):355-370. DOI: 10.1016/j.cld.2022.03.002

[7] Wiecek S, Jankowska I. Zespół Alagille'a w populacji pediatrycznej-objawy kliniczne, postępowanie diagnostyczno-terapeutyczne. Klinika Pediatryczna. 2024;**2**:2029-2047

[8] Ayoub M, Bakhsh VS, et al. Management of adults with Alagille syndrome. Hepatology International. 2023;**17**(5):1098-1112. DOI: 10.1007/s12072-023-10578-x

[9] Gilbert M, Bauer R, Rajagopalan R, et al. Alagille syndrome mutation update: Comprehensive overview of JAG1 and NOTCH 2 mutation frequencies and insight into missense variant classification. Human Mutation. 2019;**40**:2197-2220. DOI: 10.1002/humu.23879

[10] Gliwicz D, Jankowska I, Socha P. Cholestaza u dzieci. Warszawa: Standardy Medyczne. Media-Press Sp.z o.o; 2022. pp. 89-93

[11] Jones E, Clement-Jones M, Wilson D. JAGGED1 expression in human embryos: Correlation with the Alagille syndrome phenotype. Journal of Medical Genetics. 2000;**37**:658-662

[12] Leonard L, Chao G, Bakar A, et al. Clinical utility gene card for: Alagille syndrome (ALGS). European Journal of Human Genetics. 2014;**22**:e1-e4. DOI: 10.1038/ejhg.2013.140

[13] Mitchell E, Gilbert M, Loomes K. Alagille syndrome. Clinics in Liver Disease. 2018;**22**(4):625-641. DOI: 10.1016/j.cld.2018.06.001

[14] Spinner N, Gilbert M, Loomes K. Alagille syndrome. Gene Reviews. Seattle (WA): University of Washington, Seattle; 1993-2023

[15] Spinner N, Colliton R, Crosnier C, et al. Jagged 1 mutations in Alagille syndrome. Human Mutation. 2001;**17**(1):18-33

[16] Vandriel S, Li L, She H, et al. The GALA study group clinical features and natural history of 1154 Alagille syndrome patients: Results from the international multicenter GALA study group. Journal of Hepatology. 2020;**73**(Suppl.

1):554-555. Poster presentation. The Digital International Liver Congress. 2020

[17] Vandriel S, Li L, She H, et al. Natural history of liver disease in a large international cohort of children with Alagille syndrome: Results from the GALA study. Hepatology. 2023;77:512-529. DOI: 10.1002/hep.32761

[18] Tummpenny P, Eliard S. Alagille syndrome: Pathogenesis, diagnosis and management. European Journal of Human Genetics. 2012;**20**(3):251-257

[19] Kamath B, Baker A, Houven R, et al. Systematic review: The epidemiology, natural history and burden of Alagille syndrome. Journal of Pediatric Gastroenterology and Nutrition. 2018;**67**(2):148-156

[20] Kohut T, Gilbert M, Loomes K. Alagille syndrome: A focused review on clinical features, genetics and treatment. Seminars in Liver Disease. 2021;**41**(4):525-537. DOI: 10.1055/s-0041-1730951

[21] Lykavieris P, Hadchouel M, Chardot C, et al. Outcome of liver disease in children with Alagille syndrome: A study of 163 patients. Gut. 2001;**49**:431-435

[22] Roberts P, Trout A, Diliman J. Nodular macroregenerative tissue as a pattern of regeneration in cholangiopathic disorders. Pediatric Radiology. 2018;**48**(7):932-940. DOI: 10.1007/s00247-018-4129-5

[23] Dedić T, Jirsa M, Keil R, et al. Alagille syndrome mimicking biliary atresia in early infancy. PLoS One. 2015;**10**(11):e0143939. DOI: 10.1371/journal.pone.0143939

[24] Andrews A, Putra J. Central hepatic regenerative nodules in Alagille syndrome: A clinicopathological review. Fetal and Pediatric Pathology. 2021;**40**(1):69-79. DOI: 10.1080/15513815.2019.1675834

[25] Schindler E, Gilbert M, Piccoli D, et al. Alagille syndrome and risk for hepatocellular carcinoma: Need for increased surveillance in adults with mild liver phenotypes. American Journal of Medical Genetics. 2021;**185**(3):719-731. DOI: 10.1002/ajmg.a.62028

[26] Beuers U, Wolters F, Elferink R. Mechanisms of pruritus in cholestasis: Understanding and treating the itch. Nature Reviews Gastroenterology and Hepatology. 2023;**20**(1):26-36. DOI: 10.1038/s41575-022-00687-7

[27] Vajro P, Ferrante L, Paolella G. Alagille syndrome: An overview. Clinics and Research in Hepatology and Gastroenterology. 2012;**36**(3):275-277. DOI: 10.1016/j.clinre.2012.03.019

[28] Kamath B, Spinner N, Emerick K, et al. Vascular anomalies in Alagille syndrome a significant cause of morbidity and mortality. Circulation. 2004;**109**:1354-1358

[29] D'Amico A, Perillo T, Cuocolo R, et al. Neuroradiological findings in Alagille syndrome. The British Journal of Radiology. 2021;**95**:20201241

[30] Cerron-Vela C, Tierradentro-Garcia L, Rimba Z, et al. Evolution of cerebrovascular imaging and associated clinical findings in children with Alagille syndrome. Neuroradiology. 2024;**66**(8):1325-1334. DOI: 10.1007/s00234-024-03316-z

[31] Lazea C, Al-Khzouz C, Sufana C, et al. Diagnosis and management of genetic causes of middle aortic syndrome in children: A comprehensive literature review. Therapeutics and Clinical

Risk Management. 2022;**16**:233-248. DOI: 10.2147/TCRM.S348366

[32] McElhinney D, Krantz J, Bason L, et al. Analysis of cardiovascular phenotype and genotype-phenotype correlation in individuals with a JAG1 mutation and/or Alagille syndrome. Circulation. 2002;**106**(20):2567-2574. DOI: 10.1161/01.cir.0000037221.45902.69

[33] Seleh M, Kamath B, Chitayat D. Alagille syndrome clinical perspectives. The Application of Clinical Genetics. 2016;**30**:75-82

[34] Kamath B, Podkameni G, Hutchinson A, et al. Renal anomalies in Alagille syndrome: A disease-defining feature. American Journal of Medical Genetics Part A. 2012;**158**:85-89

[35] Kamath B, Chen Z, Romero R, et al. Quality of life and its determinants in a multicenter cohort of children with Alagille syndrome. The Journal of Pediatrics. 2015;**167**(2):390-396. DOI: 10.1016/j.jpeds.2015.04.077

[36] Leung D, Sorensen L, Ye W, et al. Neurodevelopmental outcomes in children with inherited liver disease and native liver. JPGN. 2022;**74**:96-103. DOI: 10.1097/MPG0000000000003337

[37] Bresnahan J, Winthrop Z, Salman R, et al. Alagille syndrome: A case report highlighting dysmorphic facies, chronic illness and depression. Case Reports in Psychiatry. 2016;**ID**:1657691. DOI: org/10.1155/2016/1657691

[38] Elisofon S, Emerick K, Sinacore J, et al. Health status of patients with Alagille syndrome. Journal of Pediatric Gastroenterology and Nutrition. 2010;**51**(6):759-765. DOI: 10.1097/MPG.0b013e3181ef3771

[39] Kim B, Fulton A. The genetics and ocular findings of Alagille syndrome. Seminars in Ophthalmology. 2007;**22**:205-210. DOI: 10.1080/08820530701745108

[40] Fukumoto M, Ikeda T, Sugiyama T, et al. A case of Alagille syndrome complicated by intraocular lens subluxation and rhegmatogenous retinal detachment. Clinical Ophthalmology. 2013;**7**:1463-1465. DOI: 10.2147/OPTH.S43753

[41] Loomes K, Spino C, Goodrich N, et al. Bone density in children with chronic liver disease correlates with growth and cholestasis. Hepatology. 2019;**69**(1):245-257. DOI: 10.1002/hep.30196

[42] Rovner A, Schall J, Jawad A, et al. Rethinking growth failure in Alagille syndrome: The role of dietary intake and steatorrhea. Journal of Pediatric Gastroenterology and Nutrition. 2002;**35**(4):495-502. DOI: 10.1097/00005176-200210000-00007

[43] Bucuvalas J, Horn J, Carlsson L, et al. Growth hormone insensitivity associated with elevated circulating growth hormone- binding protein in children with Alagille syndrome and short stature. The Journal of Clinical Endocrinology and Metabolism. 1993;**76**:1477-1482. DOI: Doi.org/10.1210/jcem.76.6.8501153

[44] Berniczei-Royko A, Chalas R, Mitura I, et al. Medical and dental management of Alagille syndrome: A review. Medical Science Monitor. 2014;**24**(20):476-480. DOI: 10.12659/MSM.890577

[45] Nagasaka H, Yorrifuji T, Egawa H, et al. Evaluation of risk for atherosclerosis in Alagille syndrome and progressive familial intrahepatic cholestasis: Two congenital cholestatic diseases with different lipoprotein

metabolisms. The Journal of Pediatrics. 2005;**146**(3):329-335. DOI: 10.1016/j.jpeds.2004.10.047

[46] Menon J, Shanmugam N, Vij M, et al. Multidisciplinary management of Alagille syndrome. Journal of Multidisciplinary Healthcare. 2022;**15**:353-364. DOI: 10.2147/JMDH.5295441

[47] Ayoub M, Kamath B. Alagille syndrome diagnostic challenges and advances in management. Diagnostics. 2020;**6:10**(11):907

[48] Kamath B, Goldstein A, Howard R, et al. Maralixibat treatment response in Alagille syndrome is associated with improved health-related quality of life. The Journal of Pediatrics. 2023;**252**:68-75

[49] Shneider B, Spino C, Kamath B, et al. Impact of long-term administration of maralixibat on children with cholestasis secondary to Alagille syndrome. Hepatology Communications. 2022;**6**:1922-1933

[50] Hansen B, Vandriel S, Vig P, et al. Event-free survival of maralixibat-treated patients with Alagille syndrome compared to a real-world cohort from GALA. Hepatology. 2024;**79**:1279-1292. DOI: 10.1097/HEP.0000000000000727

[51] Sidra tul Muntaba H, Munir M, SSajid S, et al. Ileal bile acid transporter blockers for cholestatic liver disease in pediatric patients with Alagille syndrome: A systematic review and meta-analysis. Journal of Clinical Medicine. 2022;**11**:7926. DOI: doi.org/103390/jcm.11247526

[52] Duchinsky N, Aumar M, Baker A, et al. Efficacy and safety of odevixibat in patients with Alagille syndrome (ASSERT): A phase 3, double-blind, randomized, placebo-controlled trial. The Lancet Gastroenterology and Hepatology. 2024;**9**:632-645

[53] Terner-Rosenthal J et al. Maralixibat impact on concomitant medication use for the treatment of cholestatic pruritus in Alagille syndrome: Real-world experience. In: 56th Annual Meeting of the European Society for Pediatric Gastroenterology, Hepatology and Nutrition

[54] Sturm E et al. Efficacy and safety of odevixibat over 48 weeks: Pooled data from the phase 3 ASSERT and ASSERT-EXT studies in patients with Alagille syndrome. In: 56th Annual Meeting of the European Society for Pediatric Gastroenterology, Hepatology and Nutrition.

[55] Himes R, Rosenthal P, Dilwali N, et al. Real-world experience of maralixibat in Alagille syndrome: Novel findings outside of clinical trials. Journal of Pediatric Gastroenterology and Nutrition. 2024;**78**(3):506-513. DOI: 10.1002/jpn3.12101

[56] Shirley M. Maralixibat: First approval. Drugs. 2022;**82**(1):71-76. DOI: 10.1007/s40265-021-01649-0

[57] Gonzales E, Hardikar W, Stormon M, et al. Efficacy and safety of maralixibat treatment in patients with Alagille syndrome and cholestatic pruritus (ICONIC): A randomised phase 2 study. Lancet. 2021;**398**:1581-1592

[58] Lindström E et al. In Alagille syndrome, odevixibat elevates serum unconjugated primary bile acids in patients with pruritus relief: Post-hoc analysis of data from the randomized, placebo-controlled ASSERT study. In: 56th Annual Meeting of the European Society for Pediatric Gastroenterology, Hepatology and Nutrition

[59] Pnig K, Veyckemans F, De Kock M, et al. Hemodynamic changes in patients with Alagille's syndrome during orthotopic liver transplantation. Anesthesia and Analgesia. 1999;**89**:1137-1142

[60] Kamath B, Yin W, Miller H, et al. Outcomes of the liver transplantation for patients with Alagille syndrome: The studies of pediatric liver transplantation experience. Liver Transplantation. 2012;**18**:540-548

[61] Ebel N, Goldstein A, Howard R, et al. Health care resource utilization by patients with Alagille syndrome. The Journal of Pediatrics. 2022;**2**:1-8

[62] Kamath B, Ye W, Goodrich N, et al. Childhood liver disease research network (CHILD-ReN) outcomes of childhood cholestasis in Alagille syndrome: Results of a multicenter observational study. Hepatology Communications. 2020;**4**(3):387-398

[63] Emmerick K, Rand E, Goldmutz E, et al. Features of Alagille syndrome in 92 patients: Frequency and relations to prognosis. Hepatology. 1999;**29**(3):822-829

[64] Sokol R, Gonzales E, Kamath B, et al. Predictors of 6-year event-free survival in Alagille syndrome patients treated with maralixibat, an ileal bile acid transporter inhibitor. Hepatology. 2023;**78**:1698-1710. DOI: 10.1097/HEP.0000000000000502

Chapter 3

Biliary Tract Trauma

Winnie Long, Pratibha Vemulapalli, Alexander Sockell and Brian Gilchrist

Abstract

The biliary tract may be injured iatrogenically or via trauma. Injury to the biliary tract via cholecystectomy has increased in frequency since the transition to laparoscopic technique and is one of the most feared complications of the procedure. Injury via trauma is much rarer; nevertheless injury to this tract can lead to significant morbidity and mortality. Regardless of cause of injury, diagnosis and management of injury to this system has many overlaps. In this chapter, we will cover the etiology and diagnosis of injuries for the biliary system. We will discuss the operative management using the most modern imaging and operative techniques in the setting of the Bismuth-Strasberg classification of biliary injury.

Keywords: iatrogenic, accidental, trauma, injury, gallbladder, extrahepatic

1. Introduction

The biliary tract is critical in digestion and directs bile flow for the breakdown and absorption of lipids. Cholecystectomies are one of the most common surgeries performed, often for complications of gallstones, including symptomatic cholelithiasis and cholecystitis, and less frequently, in situations of trauma. Patients are generally expected to recover to their functional baseline after removal of the gallbladder. In contrast, the biliary ducts are much more critical for normal digestive function, and injury to these ducts, whether traumatically or iatrogenically, can lead to significant morbidity and mortality. Regardless of etiology of injury, the surgical principles of repair are the same. Bile flow is redirected to allow for medical optimization before definitive repair, and the repair itself is guided by the degree and anatomy of the injury.

2. Traumatic injury to the gallbladder

Traumatic injury to the biliary tract and gallbladder is very rare, accounting for 0.1% of trauma and is commonly associated with other intra-abdominal injuries, including the liver, pancreas, and duodenum [1, 2]. Gallbladder injuries specifically are seen in approximately 3% of exploratory laparotomies in blunt trauma and are more common than common bile duct injuries [1].

The gallbladder is naturally protected by its surrounding anatomy. The costal margin and the gallbladder's recessed position lateral to the vertebral column provide a bony defense against external forces, while the kidney and liver offer visceral shields (**Figure 1**). Therefore traumatic injury to the gallbladder often presents along with additional abdominal injuries, such as injury to the liver, duodenum, and the nearby vascular structures.

Penetrating trauma is the more common form of injury and is easier to diagnose. Penetrating trauma to the abdomen needs to be explored, and during exploration, the gallbladder must be inspected clearly. In penetrating injury, there is rarely time for radiologic imaging unless the patient is stable.

In contrast, the diagnosis of gallbladder injury may be missed in blunt trauma, especially when the gallbladder alone is injured, although this is rare [3, 4]. The correct preoperative diagnosis is seldom made in this situation. The signs of gallbladder injury in this setting, as in blunt injury to the extrahepatic ducts, can be insidious and slow, especially if the bile is sterile initially or if other injuries obfuscate the issue.

When indicated, work-up may include a hepatobiliary scintigraphy scan and paracentesis (**Figure 2**). In paracentesis, a positive tap for bile can indicate biliary injury. In comparison, hepatobiliary scans are preferred for detection of more minor leaks, however, the utility is limited to hemodynamically stable patients due to the long scan times. In general, in the setting of penetrating injury, diagnosis is made at the operating table, and bile found in the abdomen necessitates careful inspection of the entire biliary system, which may be assisted with an intraoperative cholangiogram.

2.1 Classification and management of gallbladder injuries

Injuries to the gallbladder can be divided into contusion, avulsion, laceration, and acute cholecystitis [3].

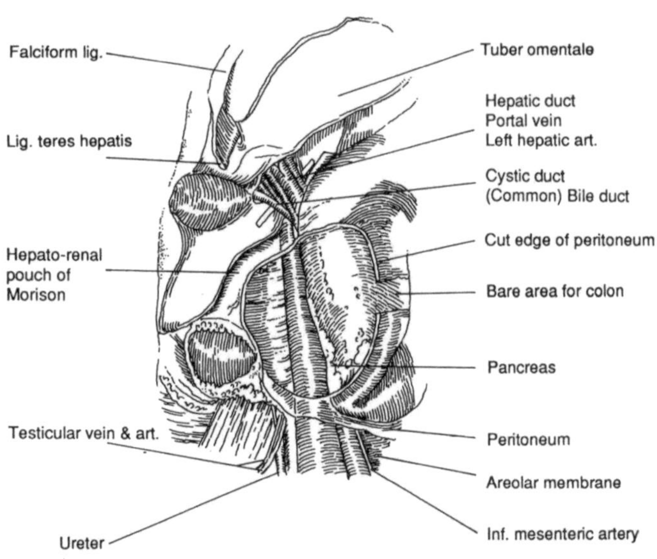

Figure 1.
The gallbladder is rarely injured in trauma due to its recessed position and protection from adjacent structures [3].

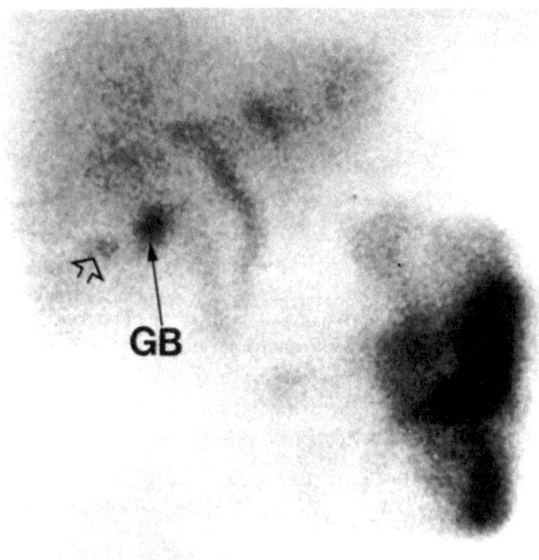

Figure 2.
This scintigraphy scan at 30 minutes reveals a small extra-biliary collection. This biloma regressed spontaneously on subsequent scans [3].

Contusion of the gallbladder is a diagnosis of exclusion. Patients may report a vague discomfort in the right upper quadrant, which may be ascribed to musculoskeletal pain. Regardless, this injury may be treated conservatively.

Avulsion occurs when a direct or shear force is applied to the closed abdominal cavity. The gallbladder is torn from its fossa and either hangs by its neck or is totally free of the liver, attached only to the common bile duct and vascular structures (**Figure 3**).

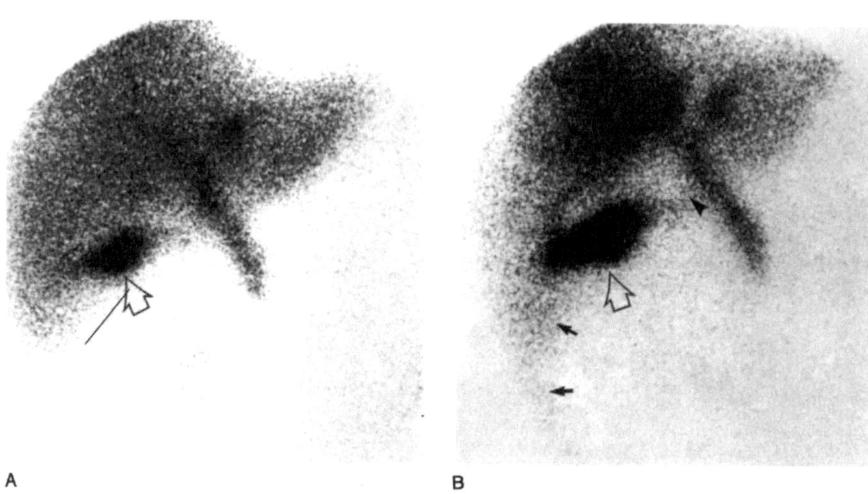

Figure 3.
(A), scintigraphy reveals a linear collection of activity (open arrow) paralleling the right hepatic margin. It is difficult to distinguish gallbladder or extravasation in this image. (B), at 45 minutes, there is increased extravasation spreading into the flank (small arrows), demonstrating extrabiliary extravasation. The source of this leak was near the cystic duct (arrowhead). This gallbladder was completely avulsed after a motor vehicle collision [3].

Laceration of the gallbladder is the most common traumatic injury to the gallbladder. However, laceration may occur with blunt trauma as well. The fundus is the most commonly lacerated area of the gallbladder.

Traumatic cholecystitis as a result of blunt abdominal trauma is a disease process that highlights the pathophysiology of typical cholecystitis. Bleeding occurs into the gallbladder either from associated liver damage or from gallbladder wall injury. Subsequently, the retained blood blocks the cystic duct, which results in distention of the gallbladder. Infection and gangrene often follow. Another factor in the development of acute cholecystitis in the trauma setting can be thrombosis of the cystic artery, with resultant ischemia of the gallbladder, though this etiology is rare.

The 2019 guidelines by the World Society of Emergency Surgery (WSES) and American Association for the Surgery of Trauma (AAST) succinctly summarizes the separate traumatic injuries to the gallbladder and biliary tract [2]. In this classification system, grades I-III describe worsening injury to the gallbladder itself, followed by progressively distal duct injuries in grades IV-V (**Table 1**).

2.2 Treatment

There are two primary approaches to gallbladder trauma, which are both predicated on hemodynamic stability: cholecystostomy and cholecystectomy. Cholecystostomy is the best option in a hemodynamically unstable patient, such as a patient with medical comorbidities or multiple traumatic injuries. A cholecystotomy tube may be quickly placed and secured with a pursestring suture to allow for drainage of the gallbladder tree. Further definitive management can then be delayed until the patient is stable and medically optimized.

For stable patients with trauma to the gallbladder, cholecystectomy is the gold standard procedure in the trauma setting. Often it is easy to perform given the premorbid state of the usually young, healthy patient. Its removal ensures that no compromised tissue remains. Whenever there is any question of occult damage to the gallbladder, it should be removed.

Grade	Description of injury
I	Gallbladder contusion/hematoma
	Portal triad contusion
II	Partial gallbladder avulsion; cystic duct intact
	Laceration or perforation of gallbladder
III	Complete gallbladder avulsion
	Cystic duct laceration
IV	Partial/complete right/left hepatic duct laceration
	Partial (<50%) common hepatic or common bile duct laceration
V	Transection of common hepatic or common bile duct (>50%)
	Combined left and right hepatic duct injuries
	Intraduodenal or intrapancreatic bile duct injuries

Table 1.
AAST Extrahepatic Biliary Tree Injuries as adapted from Coccolini et al.: Duodenopancreatic and extrahepatic biliary tree trauma:WSES-AAST guidelines. World Journal of Emergency Surgery: WJES, 14(1) [2].

The prognosis of patients who have suffered gallbladder trauma is predicated on their associated injuries. If gallbladder injuries are recognized and treated expeditiously, and there are no other serious injuries, then the prognosis is excellent.

3. Traumatic injury to the extrahepatic biliary ducts

Traumatic rupture of the duct system is related invariably to traffic accidents and may be associated with the use of seatbelts; however the mechanism of injury has never been elucidated clearly [3]. It is most certainly a shearing force, but it is a force that spares the vascular conduits while preferentially disrupting the biliary tract. When the force is great enough, the vascular structures are indeed torn, but these patients do not survive their initial injury. Disruption most often takes place at the suprapancreatic area, at the junction of the pancreas, and the common bile duct.

Ideally, repair should be immediate, but, given the usual circumstances of such an injury, such as other life-threatening problems, the safest approach is to tag the ducts' ends and place tubes in them secured with a pursestring suture, which are brought out exteriorly. Immediate anastomosis is not indicated because the ducts' ends are usually devascularized by the injury.

4. Iatrogenic trauma to the extrahepatic biliary ducts

The biliary tract is most commonly injured iatrogenically, often during a laparoscopic cholecystectomy. Since the transition to laparoscopic technique, the rate of biliary tract injury has increased (0.4–0.6% compared to open at 0.2–0.3%) [5, 6]. The rate of laparoscopic injury was at first attributed to the learning curve in laparoscopy; however, this increased rate of injury has persisted. Laparoscopic biliary injuries present earlier compared to open biliary injuries, and are associated with persistent bile leaks and concomitant vascular injury [5].

4.1 Prevention of iatrogenic injury

The risk of iatrogenic injury can be attributed to anatomic variations of the biliary tree and severe inflammation in the operating field due to the nature of the pathology, for example, in the setting of acute cholecystitis, acute biliary pancreatitis, or Mirizzi syndrome [5]. Iatrogenic injury is most often caused by misidentification of the structures, where the operator mistakes other nearby structures for the cystic artery and duct. In addition, the many variants of normal anatomy found in the biliary tree further complicate the identification of the critical structures.

The critical view of safety is a well developed concept to ensure the identification of the proper structures prior to transection (**Figure 4**). Prior to the transection of any structures, the borders of the triangle of Calot must be identified- the common hepatic duct, the cystic duct, and the liver. However, the critical view of safety may be difficult to achieve in cases with severe inflammation and fibrosis, for example, in cases of severe cholecystitis.

The 2018 Tokyo Guidelines put forth a series of recommendations to maximize safety during a laparoscopic cholecystectomy and prevent bile duct injury. In their analysis, it was noted that surgery performed within 72 hours of onset of acute

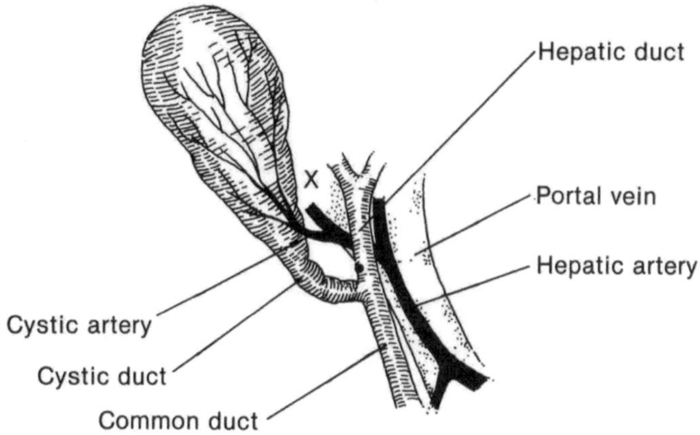

Figure 4.
Calot's triangle demarcates critical structures that must be identified before proceeding with transection of the cystic artery and duct.

cholecystitis limits the opportunity for inflammation and fibrosis to take hold and was thereby associated with fewer complications [7].

With regard to establishing the critical view of safety, consideration should be made to perform needle decompression if a distended gallbladder interferes with the view. In addition, as with surgical technique for many surgeries, effective retraction and countertraction is essential for exposure and safe dissection. Particularly critical in the dissection of Calot's triangle is the limitation of the use of electrocautery and clips. Rather, applying pressure is preferred to obtain hemostasis if bleeding is minor.

When aberrant anatomy is encountered or the critical view of safety is difficult to obtain, intraoperative cholangiography may be employed to confirm anatomy, with consideration of drain placement to aid in early detection of biliary leak. Other considerations in a case with difficult dissection include conversion of the standard laparoscopic approach to bailout procedures, including open conversion, subtotal cholecystectomy, or cholecystostomy. Whether to convert to open is heavily dependent on the surgeon's experience performing open procedures. In comparison, subtotal cholecystectomy is a bailout option that can be performed in either laparoscopic or open cases. Of note, laparoscopic subtotal cholecystectomy has been associated with increased postoperative bile leakage compared to open technique; however, compared to open technique, laparoscopic subtotal cholecystectomy is associated with lower rates of bile duct injury, postoperative complications, reoperation, and mortality [7].

4.2 Clinical presentation

Biliary duct injuries manifest themselves over a period of 2 weeks to 2 months. Jaundice, which may be intermittent, biliary fistulization through the wound, alcoholic stools, and darkened urine indicate the diagnosis. Although these symptoms would be clear indication of a biliary leak, the clinical presentation may be more insidious, with patients complaining of vague abdominal pain or distension, nausea, vomiting, or ileus [8]. Here a high index of suspicion for injury, and the utilization of various imaging techniques aids in the diagnosis and surgical planning.

4.3 Imaging

Ultrasound is often the first diagnostic study in the evaluation of the biliary tree and gallbladder because it is affordable, quick, and easy to perform. This allows for assessment of dilation of the biliary ducts and for fluid collections in the region. With the addition of a Doppler evaluation, the operator can concurrently assess for associated vascular injuries. However, assessment of a fluid collection can be equivocal on ultrasound, in which case a computed tomography scan can be utilized to better define the fluid collection and associated vascular injuries with improved sensitivity to 96% compared to 70% via ultrasound (**Figure 5**) [9]. Regardless, neither of these studies can reliably distinguish the type of fluid collection, whether it is a biloma, hematoma, seroma, or abscess [10].

Magnetic resonance cholangiopancreatography (MRCP) and hepatobiliary scintigraphy scans provide a more detailed noninvasive assessment of the biliary tree. According to the 2020 World Society of Emergency Surgery (WSES) guidelines for the detection and management of bile duct injury, the gold standard study for detection of biliary leak is MRCP as it provides excellent noninvasive visualization of the extrahepatic biliary ducts [10]. If combined with dynamic contrast-enhanced magnetic resonance using a hepatocyte-selective contrast with biliary excretion, the functional anatomy and patency of the biliary tree can additionally be assessed, leading to a detection rate nearing 100% [10]. However, in institutions where a hepatocyte-selective contrast is not available, MRCP has the potential to miss small leaks as MRCP alone does not evaluate the path of bile flow [8]. In such cases, scintigraphy is the optimal noninvasive method to assess biliary tree function. Of note, the spatial resolution of the bile ducts in scintigraphy scans is poor, but detection of abnormal bile flow alone may be enough to prompt a clinician to seek further invasive

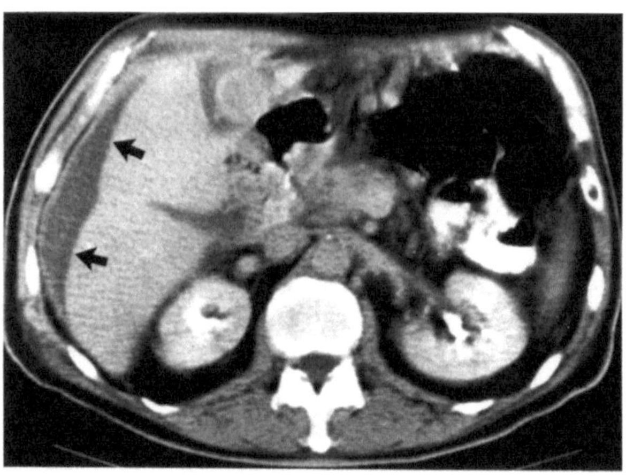

Figure 5.
Computed tomography scan demonstrating a post-traumatic fluid collection. At this level of the scan, this may represent a subcapsular hematoma, biloma, or abscess [3].

studies that can not only diagnose but also treat the pathology, such as an endoscopic retrograde cholangiopancreatography (ERCP) or percutaneous transhepatic cholangiography (PTC) [10].

4.4 Classification

The discussion of management of biliary injury is best achieved by first classifying the type of injury. The most common stratification of biliary injury is the Bismuth-Strasberg classification. The Bismuth system focuses on lesions to the common hepatic duct, where increasing grading is associated with progressively proximal lesions towards the hepatic confluence. In comparison, the Strasberg classification adds other minor injuries to the Bismuth system that do not involve full transection of the ductal system, including lesions to the cystic duct and right hepatic duct (**Table 2**, **Figure 6**).

4.5 Management of extrahepatic biliary injuries

Management of extrahepatic biliary injuries is directed by degree of injury. Once an injury is recognized by noninvasive imaging, ERCP and PTC are excellent minimally invasive options to diagnose and treat low-grade and low-output leaks (ie Strasberg A-D injuries) [5, 10]. ERCP is more likely to succeed in extrahepatic injuries with a defect of <5 mm and without associated abscesses and bilomas [10]. When a leak is identified with ERCP, the operator may place a stent and perform a sphincterotomy to decrease the pressure gradient in the biliary system [10]. The stents are left in situ for 4–8 weeks and removed if retrograde cholangiography shows resolution of the leak.

Even in high-grade leaks (ie Strasberg E1-E4 injuries), stent placement with ERCP can be utilized as a temporizing measure to optimize the operating field before definitive surgery [9]. Similarly, percutaneous transhepatic drains can be utilized as a temporizing measure to redirect bile flow prior to definitive management [9]. Although these interventions have the ability to both diagnose and treat a bile leak simultaneously, they are not necessarily recommended as first-line for diagnosis, as

Biliary anatomy	Bismuth	Strasberg
Cystic duct leak or leak from small ducts in liver bed	–	A
Occlusion of aberrant RHD	–	B
Transection without ligation of an aberrant RHD	–	C
Lateral injury to CBD (<50% circumference)	–	D
CHD stricture, stump >2 cm	Type 1	E1
CHD stricture, stump <2 cm	Type 2	E2
Hilar stricture, no residual CHD, preserved confluence	Type 3	E3
Hilar stricture, involvement of confluence, loss of communication between RHL and LHL	Type 4	E4
Stricture of low-lying right sectorial duct (alone or with concomitant common hepatic duct stricture)	Type 5	E5

RHD: right hepatic duct; LHD: left hepatic duct; CHD: common hepatic duct; CBD: common bile duct.

Table 2.
Bismuth-Strasberg Classifications of Biliary Injury, as adapted from Mohkam et al., Post-cholecystectomy biliary injury. Liver, Gall Bladder, and Bile Ducts [5].

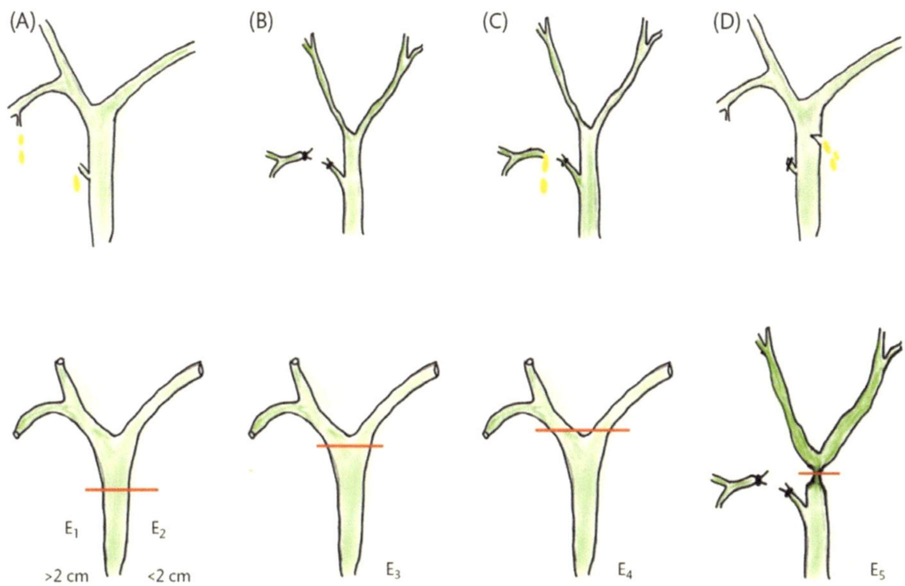

Figure 6.
As reproduced from Mohkam et al., Post-cholecystectomy biliary injury. Liver, Gall Bladder, and Bile Ducts [5].

they are invasive and are associated with significant complications, including pancreatitis, bleeding, and cholangitis [10].

5. Operative management

Definitive repair of a biliary leak should first proceed with an intraoperative cholangiogram to clearly delineate the anatomy and biliary lesions. In a study of bile duct injuries during laparoscopic cholecystectomy, 84% of reconstructions were successful in the first attempt with utilization of a cholangiogram [11].

There are three classically described operative injuries to the biliary ducts: axial, partial transverse division, and complete transverse division.

5.1 Axial wounds

Large ducts should be repaired longitudinally with a single-layered closure of absorbable suture (**Figure 7**). Two-layered anastomoses increase the risk of duct obstruction due to the inversion of tissue, and nonabsorbable sutures can find their way into the lumen and become a nidus for the precipitation of bile [11]. Small ducts, on the other hand, should be repaired transversely via the Heineke-Mikulicz technique (**Figure 8**).

5.2 Partial transverse division

Generally, in a partial transverse injury, it is the anterior wall of the biliary duct that is involved. Repair is facilitated by the temporary placement of a stent. Retrieval of the stent is aided by placing a suture through the stent before it is positioned in the

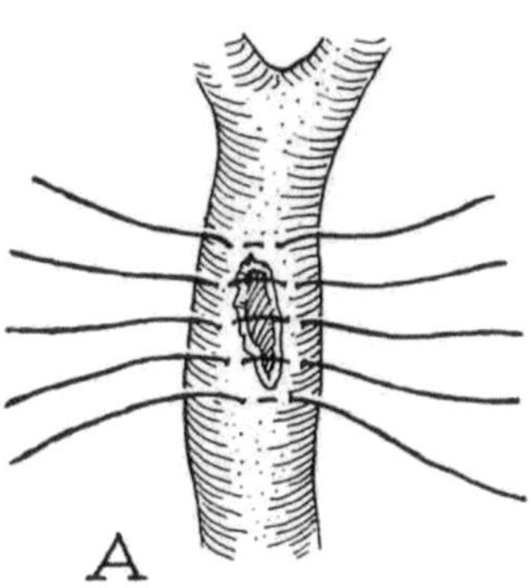

Figure 7.
Long-axial closure of an incised common duct by single tier suture. All of the sutures are place (A) before any are tied (B) [3].

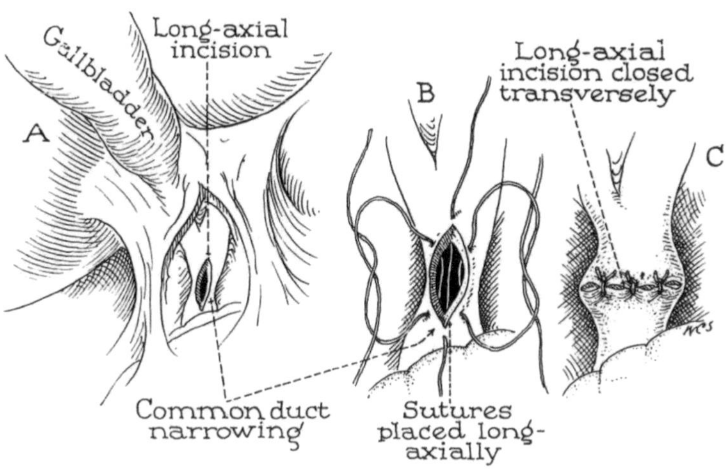

Figure 8.
The Heineke-Mikulicz technique ensures patency of the duct [3].

biliary tract. Transverse suturing of the defect is begun using through-and-through sutures that are left untied until the stent is removed (**Figure 9**). An alternative approach is the use of a T tube as a stent and removing the T tube through a separate site away from the injury, which obviates the potential for disruption of the repair at the time of removal.

5.3 Complete transverse division

For high-grade biliary injuries with complete transection of the biliary ducts, surgical intervention with hepaticojejunostomy is required. As opposed to an end-to-end repair, there is decreased tension on a hepaticojejunostomy, which thereby decreases the rate of postoperative strictures [8]. When the distance between the biliary convergence and the stump is greater or equal to 2 cm (Strasberg E1), a standard hepaticojejunostomy using a Roux-en-Y loop can be performed. If the stump is less than 2 cm or more proximal (Strasberg E2-E3), the Hepp-Couinaud technique is preferred [5]. The Hepp-Couinaud technique takes advantage of the

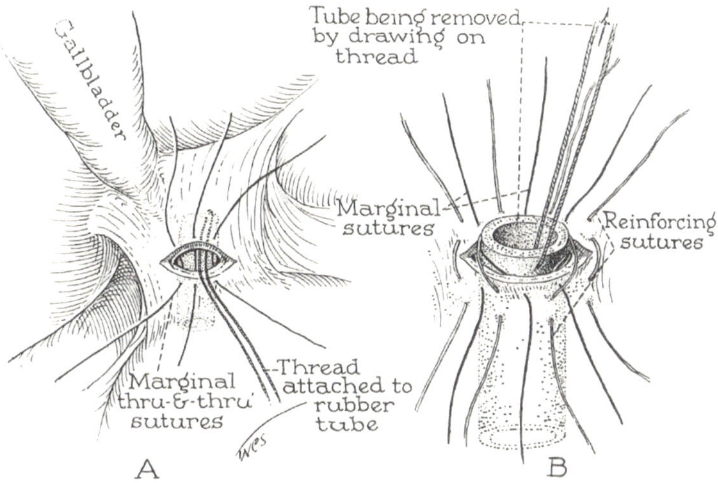

Figure 9.
Repair of partial transverse injury by suturing over a stent. A, sutures placed over the stent are inserted in the duct. B, the tube is removed before sutures are tied.

long and horizontal anatomy of the left bile duct. In this repair, the hilar plate is lowered, and the left bile duct is dissected so that the surgeon can perform a latero-lateral anastomosis with a Roux-en-Y loop using interrupted absorbable 4–0 or 5–0 sutures (**Figure 10**). Finally, if the biliary convergence is disrupted, the surgeon often will need to perform multiple biliodigestive anastomoses onto the Roux-en-Y (**Figure 11**). Patients should be medically optimized for these repairs by redirecting bile flow to allow inflammation to abate. Definitive repair should be performed by a hepatobiliary surgeon.

Bile duct injury is concomitantly associated with vascular injury in 16.7–47% of cases and most often involves the right hepatic artery due to its proximity to the common hepatic duct [8, 12]. Isolated occlusion of this artery is usually well tolerated in patients due to collateral flow through the hilar marginal artery and hilar plexus [5, 8, 12]. However, in the setting of injury to the bile duct, injury of the right hepatic artery increases the risk of postoperative stricture and liver ischemia [12]. Repair of the right hepatic artery may be attempted, but the opportunity to repair is limited because repair must be performed within hours of the injury and because the injury is often too severe for repair. These right hepatic artery injuries are more

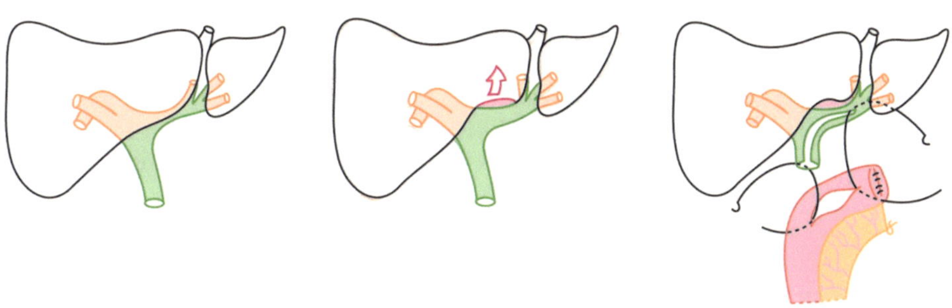

Figure 10.
Hepp-Couinaud technique, as reproduced from Mohkam et al., Post-cholecystectomy biliary injury. Liver, Gall Bladder, and Bile Ducts [5].

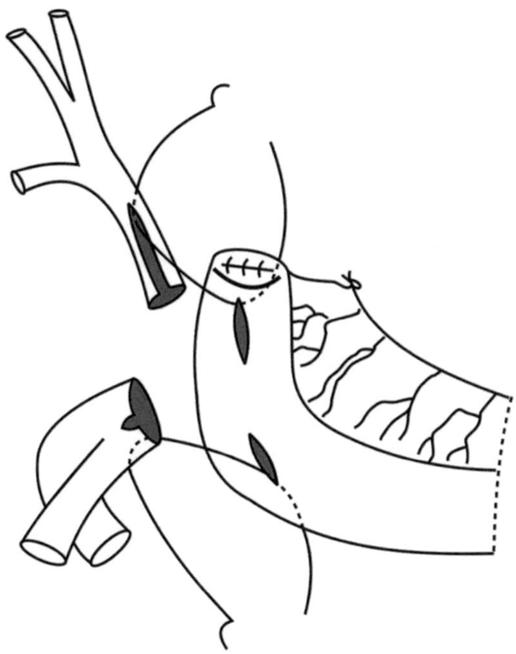

Figure 11.
The right and left hepatic ducts anastomosed separately on a single Roux-en-Y loop, as reproduced from Mohkam et al., Post-cholecystectomy biliary injury. Liver, Gall Bladder, and Bile Ducts [5].

often managed expectantly by monitoring for hepatic ischemia and secondary biliary cirrhosis. Should either of these develop, the patient may require liver resection or transplantation [5, 8].

5.4 Operative approach

The open approach has been the gold standard for repair of biliary duct injuries; however, this approach is associated with increased morbidity, ranging from rates from 10 to 42.9% [13]. Laparoscopic technique is associated with decreased morbidity but may prove challenging in certain patients. Laparoscopic technique may be considered in more straightforward repairs; however, if the injury proves to be complex, the duct is small (<3 mm) or port positioning is difficult, the open approach may be preferred [14]. Alternatively, a robotic approach improves the magnification of the small operative field and improves range of motion without the morbidity of an open surgery. However, both the laparoscopic and robotic approaches in definitive bile duct repair must be studied more extensively. Thus far, a retrospective comparative study in 2019 found comparative results between robotic and laparoscopic approaches to bile duct reconstruction, with similar blood losses, operative times, and recovery times [13].

6. Morbidity and mortality

Injury to the biliary tract is associated with significant morbidity and mortality. Patients with common bile duct injury have increased mortality of 7.2% and

14.5% at 1 year and 5 years, respectively, compared to the general population [5, 6]. The morbidity and mortality is related to the severity of injury, as injuries requiring surgical reconstruction are associated with many complications from the repair. Severe injuries are associated with postoperative biloma and acute cholecystitis or cholangitis at the time of operation [6]. The most significant complication after surgical reconstruction of the injury is cholangitis in up to 10% of cases [11]. This is followed by anastomotic leak and abdominal abscesses. Up to 11% of patients require reintervention, though most can be managed percutaneously or endoscopically [5]. Important factors to reducing the morbidity of these injuries is related to early recognition and referral to a hepatobiliary surgeon for repair [8, 11].

Factors at play for the optimal timing of repair include time of diagnosis and the time required to optimize the patient for reconstruction. If an iatrogenic injury is discovered intraoperatively, a hepatobiliary surgeon should be consulted immediately. Attempts to repair the lesion without a hepatobiliary expertise has shown to have success rates as low as 17% [6]. Rather, the primary surgeon should place drains for biliary diversion and transfer to a tertiary care center. However, if the leak is discovered outside the operating room, or occurs in the setting of trauma, the surrounding structures are often inflamed, either from the pre-existing condition, such as cholecystitis, or simply from exposure to bile. Such patients should have bile flow re-directed (i.e. via percutaneous drains), and any intra-abdominal infections must be fully treated to optimize the operative field for reconstruction [11]. Furthermore, in the case of concomitant vascular injury, delaying reconstruction allows for delineation of ischemia. The optimal timing for repair is therefore multifactorial and therefore controversial. Overall, the timing has not shown to impact severe postoperative complications, re-interventions, or mortality [6].

7. Conclusion

Injuries to the biliary tract are difficult to diagnose due to nonspecific symptoms on presentation and are associated with high rates of morbidity and mortality. The approach to management of gallbladder trauma is relatively straightforward. Stable patients should undergo a cholecystectomy whereas unstable patients should be diverted with a cholecystostomy.

In extrahepatic biliary injury, a high index of suspicion is required in trauma settings and status post biliary surgeries for early diagnosis. Imaging studies are critical in the workup of a biliary tract injury. Ultrasound is a low-cost and effective study to initially assess for fluid collections. For evaluation of a leak and for clearer delineation of the biliary tree, the gold standard imaging is MRCP with hepatocyte-selective contrast; however in institutions where this is unavailable, a hepatobiliary scintigraphy is next study of choice, though spatial resolution is limited in this scan.

Minor injuries (ie Strasberg A-D) are best managed with ERCP with sphincterotomy and stent placement. In high grade injuries (ie Strasberg E1-E4), ERCP and PTC can be utilized to divert biliary flow and serve as a temporizing measure until the patient is medically optimized for definitive repair.

For best patient outcome, operative repair should be conducted by an experienced hepatobiliary surgeon as soon as the patient is medically stable. Partial injuries may be repaired primarily or over a stent; however, high grade injuries should be repaired with a hepaticojejunostomy. The current gold standard for these repairs are via the open approach, though new studies suggest that laparoscopic and robotic technique may be utilized with decreased morbidity compared to open.

Author details

Winnie Long*, Pratibha Vemulapalli, Alexander Sockell and Brian Gilchrist
The Brooklyn Hospital Center, Brooklyn, NY, USA

*Address all correspondence to: wlong@tbh.org

References

[1] Mirza A, Filobbos R, Kausar A, O'Reilly DA. Injury to the liver, pancreas, spleen, gallbladder, and extra-hepatic bile duct. In: Abdominal Trauma, Peritoneum, and Retroperitoneum. Oxford, UK: Oxford University Press; 2022. pp. 21-40. Available from: https://academic.oup.com/book/44587/chapter/377368421 [Accessed: 4 May 2024]

[2] Coccolini F, Kobayashi L, Kluger Y, Moore EE, Ansaloni L, Biffl W, et al. Duodeno-pancreatic and extrahepatic biliary tree trauma: WSES-AAST guidelines. World Journal of Emergency Surgery: WJES. 2019;**14**(1):1-23. Available from: /pmc/articles/PMC6907251/shacke [Accessed: 17 May 2024]

[3] Gilchrist BF, Trunkey DD. Biliary tract trauma. In: Zuidema GD, editor. Shackelford's Surgery of the Alimentary Tract. 4th ed. Philadelphia: WB Saunders Company; 1996. pp. 338-354

[4] Longmire WP, McArthur MS. Occult injuries of the liver, bile duct, and pancreas after blunt abdominal trauma. The American Journal of Surgery. 1973;**125**(6):661-666

[5] Mohkam K, Mabrut JY, Rode A, Lesurtel M. Post-cholecystectomy biliary injury. In: Liver, Gall Bladder, and Bile Ducts. Oxford, UK: Oxford University Press; 2023. pp. 366-C33P110. Available from: https://academic.oup.com/book/54239/chapter/422455979 [Accessed 11 May 2024]

[6] Conde Monroy D, Torres Gómez P, Rey Chaves CE, Recamán A, Pardo M, Sabogal JC. Early versus delayed reconstruction for bile duct injury a multicenter retrospective analysis of a hepatopancreaticobiliary group. Scientific Reports. 2022;**12**(1):11609. Available from: /pmc/articles/PMC9270444/ [Accessed: 26 May 2024]

[7] Wakabayashi G, Iwashita Y, Hibi T, Takada T, Strasberg SM, Asbun HJ, et al. Tokyo guidelines 2018: Surgical management of acute cholecystitis: Safe steps in laparoscopic cholecystectomy for acute cholecystitis (with videos). Journal of Hepato-Biliary-Pancreatic Sciences. 2018;**25**(1):73-86. Available from: https://pubmed.ncbi.nlm.nih.gov/29095575/ [Accessed: 7 June 2024]

[8] Lau WY, Lai ECH, Lau SHY. Management of bile duct injury after laparoscopic cholecystectomy: A review. ANZ Journal of Surgery. 2010;**80**(1-2):75-78. Available from: https://onlinelibrary.wiley.com/doi/full/10.1111/j.1445-2197.2009.05205.x [Accessed: 12 May 2024]

[9] Bharathy KGS, Negi SS. Postcholecystectomy bile duct injury and its sequelae: Pathogenesis, classification, and management. Indian Journal of Gastroenterology. 2014;**3**(3):201-215. Available from: https://link.springer.com/article/10.1007/s12664-013-0359-5 [Accessed: 12 May 2024]

[10] de' Angelis N, Catena F, Memeo R, Coccolini F, Martínez-Pérez A, Romeo OM, et al. 2020 WSES guidelines for the detection and management of bile duct injury during cholecystectomy. World Journal of Emergency Surgery. 2021;**16**(1):1-27. Available from: https://wjes.biomedcentral.com/articles/10.1186/s13017-021-00369-w [Accessed: 17 May 2024]

[11] Stewart L, Way LW. Bile duct injuries during laparoscopic cholecystectomy:

Factors that influence the results of treatment. Archives of Surgery. 1995;**130**(10):1123-1128. Available from: https://jamanetwork.com/journals/jamasurgery/fullarticle/596351 [Accessed: 2 June 2024]

[12] Strasberg SM, Scott HW. An analytical review of vasculobiliary injury in laparoscopic and open cholecystectomy. HPB Journal. 2010;**13**:1-14

[13] Cuendis-Velázquez A, Trejo-Ávila M, Bada-Yllán O, Cárdenas-Lailson E, Morales-Chávez C, Fernández-Álvarez L, et al. A new era of bile duct repair: Robotic-assisted versus laparoscopic Hepaticojejunostomy. Journal of Gastrointestinal Surgery. 2019;**23**(3):451-459

[14] Gupta V, Jayaraman S. Role for laparoscopy in the management of bile duct injuries. Canadian Journal of Surgery. 2017;**60**(5):300. Available from: /pmc/articles/PMC5608577/ [Accessed: 5 July 2024]

Chapter 4

Diagnostic and Treatment Role of Choledochoscope for Laparoscopic and Open Bile Duct Surgery

Sotirov Dobromir Yordanov and Petar Filev

Abstract

The aim of this study is to assess the feasibility of intraoperative cholangioscopy for diagnostic and therapeutic purposes during laparoscopic and open bile duct exploration in patients with acute cholecystitis. From 2021 to 2024, 32 patients – 15 men and 17 women – with mean age of 76 years were admitted with acute cholecystitis and choledocholithiasis. A total of 27 patients were operated by laparoscopy and 5 patients by open surgery. Intraoperative cholangioscopy (IOCs) was attempted in all patients and was successful. Intraoperative choledochoscopy was successfully performed in all 32 patients. The mean duration of this examination was 20 min [15–55]. Extraction of common bile duct stones was achieved by laparoscopic approach in 27 patients and by open exploration of CBD in 5 patients. All laparoscopic interventions were finished by the placement of a T-tube into the common bile duct with no complications of infection or bile leakage. Post exploratory T-tube cholangiography was a routine procedure on the 21st day after the procedure. After confirmation of no residual stones in the CBD, the T-tube was removed. Laparoscopic IOCs is a reliable and safe diagnostic and therapeutic method for CBD stones even for complicated cases of acute cholecystitis.

Keywords: acute cholecystits, choledocholithiasis, laparoscopic approach, common bile duct exploration, surgery

1. Introduction

Cholangioscopy or choledochoscopy is defined as an endoscopic procedure, which allows direct intraductal visualization of the biliary tree. In the setting of multiple biliary diseases, this different approach proposes diagnostic and therapeutic resolution of many issues.

The introduction of choledoscopy started back in 1887 when Thornton described two successful cases in which common bile duct stones were removed *via* a dilated cystic duct. In 1890, Courvoisier described an operation for retrieving a retained stone [1, 2].

In 1937, Babcock Hollenberg and Eikner, each working independently, used a cystoscope to remove gallstones through a cholecystotomy [3]. The development of the first modern rigid choledochoscope should be accorded to Monroe McIver in 1941 when he modified the cystoscope, 5 mm in diameter with a right angle 7 cm from the tip. Since that time, no significant work was published until Wildegans reported his experience with his new scope at the Surgical Conference in Berlin in 1953 [3–6].

The first flexible scope with better maneuver¬ability and flexibility was introduced by Shore and Lippman in 1965 who reported a series of 100 patients [14]. Subsequently, Hopkins developed a special rod lens system, which was integrated into the rigid choledochoscope [7]. In the 1970s, Olympus introduced the new series of choledochoscopes with improved fiber optics and maneuverability. These flexible choledochoscopes were gradually improved and modified by Ashby up to now [17]. Today, the modern flexible fiber optic system is ultrasmall with high resolution providing a clear image [1, 8, 9].

The new modern device has an irrigation channel that by injection of saline solution produces distention and clearing of the bile ducts. This water medium helps with easier advancement of cholangioscope. The working channel of modern choledochoscope has the advantage to allow insertion of different accessories (e.g., Dormia basket, biopsy forceps, cholangio-catheter, Fogarty catheter) needed for different operative procedures—stone extraction, biopsy, and dilation of papilla.

These days, the introduction of cholangioscope can be performed through different approaches: endoscopic peroral, percutaneous transhepatic, intraoperative transcystic or transcholedochal. Endoscopic peroral access is the most frequently utilized approach today. This endoscopic technique is part of endoscopic retrograde cholangiopancreatography/ERCP and allows the advancement of cholangioscope through the duodenoscope and the papilla of Vateri. Example for this access is the Spyglass cholangioscope (Boston Scientific, USA). There is a different approach where we can access the CBD with choledochoscope by peroral route without duodenoscope-direct peroral choledochoscopy. The main difference between these two accesses is the larger diameter of choledochoscope used for direct method—5.9 versus 3.6 mm for Spyglass [10].

There are the cases when the endoscopic papillary access is more complex; for instance, in resection of the stomach, we could apply Japanese percutaneous transhepatic approach. With the CHF-CB30; Olympus Medical choledochoscope the technique is riskier and more traumatic for the patient, because of the liver penetration, but allows better maneuverability in the bile ducts [10–14].

Clinical applications of cholangioscopy are versatile and used for many diagnostic and therapeutic purposes in the field of bile tract diseases.

The most common diagnostic and therapeutic application of cholangiography is the visualization and extraction of bile duct stones.

Gallstones are one of the most common digestive problems with frequency 11–36% in different populations. Between 6 and 12% of patients with gallstones have CBD stones, and this dependence increases as age increases [7, 15].

Today, we know the three different modalities for the treatment of CBD stones:

1. Laparoscopic cholecystectomy and endoscopic retrograde cholangiopancreatography (ERCP) before or after operation (LC + ERCP).

2. Conventional exploration of CBD by laparotomy and subsequent T-tube placement (CCBDE).

3. One stage laparoscopic common bile duct exploration with laparoscopic cholecystectomy (LCBDE) [16].

After the first laparoscopic cholecystectomy in 1985, the laparoscopic technique becomes more and more common with low morbidity and better outcomes in experienced hands [17].

On the other hand, today, the most popular treatment method for CBD stones is ERCP with 85–95% success rate. According to the latest ESGE guidelines, this technique is the first-line approach recommended for the treatment of bile stones [18, 19].

Although the ERCP is a highly efficient approach, there are difficult cases. The remaining 10–15% of retained stones after ERCP are challenging to remove and require different approach. The characteristics of these difficult bile duct stones are as follows [10]:

1. Size of a stone larger than 15 mm.

2. Multiple stones or square-shaped stones.

3. Location in the intrahepatic duct or in the cystic duct.

One of the possible resolutions of this challenge is extracorporeal shock wave lithotripsy or lithotripsy assisted by cholangioscopy [10].

Even the technique is very useful in clinical practice, and we know the disadvantages of this method (up to 15% complications) [20, 21]:

1. Two-stage procedure.

2. Risk of complications (e.g., acute pancreatitis, hemorrhage, and duodenal perforation).

3. In the long term, accomplished papillosphincterotomy predisposes to malfunction of papilla, chronic inflammation of CBD, and biliary tract cancer.

On the other hand, despite expectation of many surgeons, LCBDE was less preferred in the past because of the lack of experience. Today, the technique has many benefits according to different authors [22, 23]:

1. Single-stage procedure.

2. Less complications than ERCP or CCBDE.

3. Keeps the normal function of papilla.

Comparing the two different methods—ERCP and LCBDE, Kharbutli et al. reported that one-stage management of symptomatic CBDS is associated with less morbidity and mortality (7 and 0.19%) than two-stage management (13.5 and 0.5%) [24, 25].

Recently, the study of 14 randomized controlled trials with included 2181 patients has been published. In this study, authors compare the efficacy and safety of LC-LCBDE and ERCP-LC. The results show no difference between the two groups in terms of surgical success, stone clearance, retained stones, operation time, and total morbidity. LC-LCBDE had a higher rate of bile leakage, but ERCP-LC had a higher rate of postoperative pancreatitis, cholangitis and hemorrhage. The conclusion is that both methods are safe, effective, and minimally invasive for the treatment of CBD stones [26].

According to different studies, the most common complications after LCBDE are as follows:

1. T-tube dislocation.

2. Bile leakage.

3. Pancreatitis and infection.

4. Bleeding.

5. Retained stones after the operation.

Conventional laparotomy with CBD exploration is a traditional access for the resolution of choledocholithiasis. Usually, the indication for this method is unsuccessful ERCP or CCBD because of fixed stone at the papilla. After stone extraction, the operation is accomplished by the placement of a T-tube into the bile duct.

Comparing the LCBDE and CCBDE, Grubnik et al. found low complication rate in laparoscopic approach (5 vs. 12.7%) [27].

After the study of Aydin based on 280 patients, it was reported that LCBDE is a more efficient technique (93 vs. 82,8%), with less hospital stays (6 days vs. 11 days), less morbidity (9 vs. 24%), less mortality rate (1,2 vs. 6%), and lower rate of wound infection (0,6 vs. 10%) compared to CCBDE. Different study also confirms the low morbidity rate after LCBDE to be around 8% [28, 29].

The most life-threatening complication after CBD exploration and T-tube placement is the dislocation of tube with bile leakage, biliary peritonitis, and need of reoperation with a high mortality rate. According to different studies, the bile leakage has been reported to be between 6 and 14.6%, biliary peritonitis between 2.5 and 19.6%, and reoperation of 4.3% [29–31].

The problem with retained stones after different extraction methods is still valid. Many authors confirm that retained stones after LCBDE are lower (6.1 vs. 17.2%) after CCBDE. These results were confirmed by other studies [29, 32].

According to the different studies, LCBDE has a high successful rate of stone extraction (93,9%). The author suggests that the main reason for that is the stone extraction through the choledochotomy access [23, 25, 29].

The advancement of the laparoscopic exploration of the CBD increases the number of diagnostic and therapeutic applications of cholangioscopy.

1. Extraction of migrated biliary stent.

2. Biopsy of benign polyps in the CBD.

3. Diagnosis of primary sclerosing cholangitis (PSC).

4. Endoscopic hemostasis in the case of post-ERCP bleeding.

5. Radiofrequency ablation (RFA) in cases of intraductal biliary lesions.

2. Patients and methods

In our study from 2021 to 2024, we included 32 patients admitted in the hospital for acute cholecystitis with confirmed gallstones (cholecystolithiases). From these admissions, there were 15 men and 17 women.

All the patients were ≥ 65 years. In this study, 21 patients were ≥ 75 years. Comorbidities were presented in 22 instances. Cardiovascular disease was presented in 18 patients, hypertension in 15, diabetes type 1 in 11 cases, diabetes type 2 in 8, renal issue in 6, and pulmonary problem in 2.

In this series, 17 patients had a previous abdominal surgery (laparotomy).

Four patients had a previous unsuccessful ERCP for bile duct stone extraction.

Each patient was evaluated for the presence of associated bile duct stones by history, physical examination, laboratory results, and imaging. Symptomatic acute cholecystitis was presented in 21 patients, cholangitis in 11, and acute pancreatitis in 13.

During the evaluation of these 32 patients, 13 were found to have cholestasis (AP and GGT) and 19 patients had increased direct bilirubin (jaundice). During the preoperative workup, 18 patients had visible stones in the CBD on the ultrasonography (US) and angio CT. MRI was complementary examination and found stones in the CBD in seven cases.

All 32 patients had a dilation of CBD ≥10 mm.

In our study, 27 patients were operated by laparoscopy and five patients were operated by open surgery (laparotomy).

If the patient has complications of gallstones (e.g., acute cholecystitis, cholangitis, acute pancreatitis, and septic complication), usually we start conservative treatment with antibiotics and infusions. After the resolution of symptoms and the patient having normal laboratory results and normal vital signs, we start the discussion about operation and estimation of operative risk.

In 11 cases, there was a pericholecystic abscess provoked by acute cholecystitis. Four patients were treated by percutaneous biliary drainage and subsequently operated by laparoscopy. Seven patients have an emergency laparoscopic operation for this pericholecystic abscess. Five patients were treated simultaneously for stones in the CBD by a choledochoscope. Two patients had an operation for stones in the bile duct 1 month after emergency cholecystectomy.

3. Results

During the evaluation of these 32 patients with cholestasis or increased direct bilirubin, seven patients had no visible stones on the US, CT, and MRI before operation, but we found them in the CBD during the exploration by the cholangioscope (**Figures 1** and **2**).

We applied laparoscopic approach for 27 patients and open surgical access for five patients.

In our series, we use the trans-cystic access in five cases and trans-choledochal approach in 27 cases.

The medium size of the extracted CBD stone was 7 mm (from 3 to 28 mm).

The number of extracted stones was 1–12.

We have applied the cholangioscope for other diagnostic and therapeutic purposes in four patients. We have made a biopsy of polyp in the CBD for one patient and an extraction of migrated biliary stent in patient with cholangitis after ERCP (**Figures 3** and **4**).

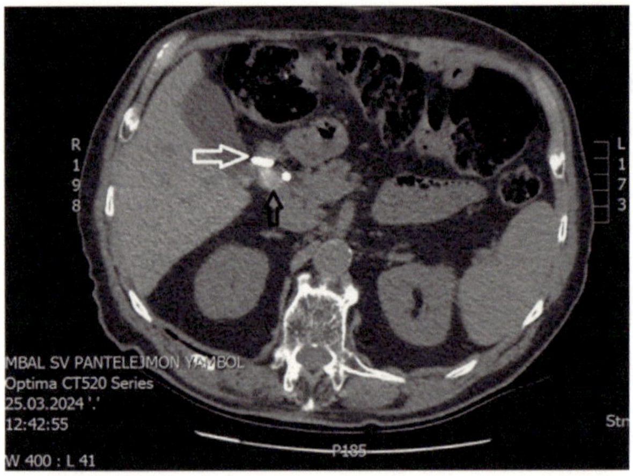

Figure 1.
Migration of biliary stent [post ERCP] with stone in the CBD.

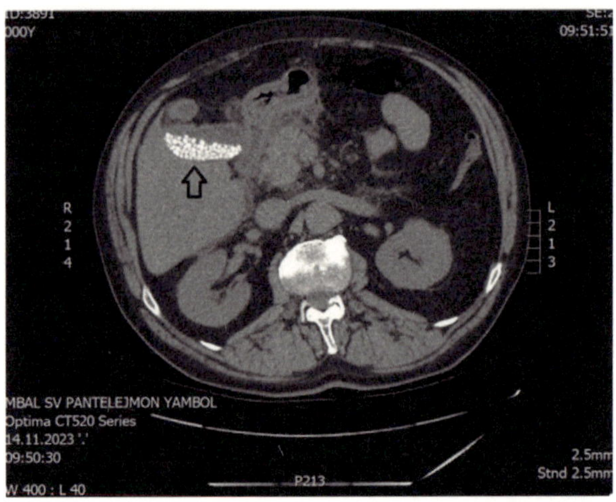

Figure 2.
Gallstones on the CT.

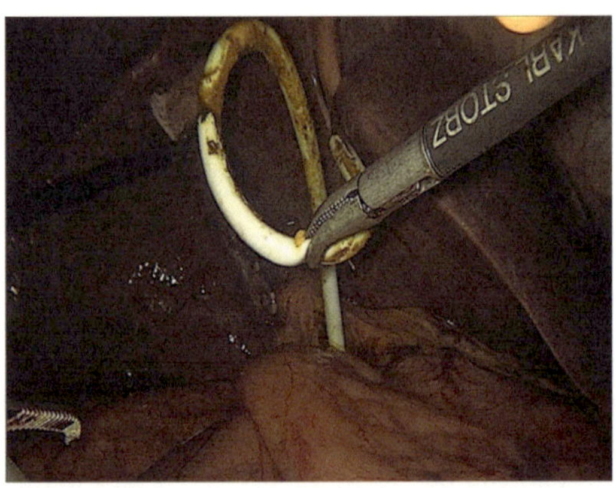

Figure 3.
Extraction of biliary stent after choledochotomy.

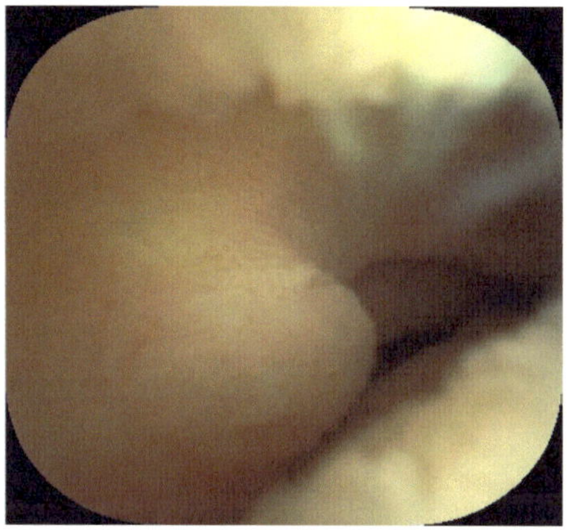

Figure 4.
Biopsy of polyp in the CBD [picture through the cholangioscope].

Two patients had biopsies—for cholangiocarcinoma and pancreatic cancer.

In our study, there was no bile leakage and no drain dislodgment or bile peritonitis in the postoperative period. There was no patient with hemorrhage or infection complication and no mortality.

4. Operative technique for cholangioscopy during laparoscopic and open surgical approach

For all patients in this series, we start the exploration of CBD by laparoscopic approach. Previous laparotomy is not a contraindication for laparoscopic access. All the operations were performed by one surgeon.

In our department for the exploration of CBD, we use two different sizes of flexible choledochoscope 3 and 5 mm/Shanghai SeeGen Photoelectric Technology Co.Ltd. – Briview. The choledochoscope ф 5.3 has 380 mm length and 2.6 mm working channel. The choledochoscope ф 3 has 580 mm length and 1.2 mm working channel.

The choice between them depends on the diameter of CBD. The flexible choledochoscope has a working channel for the introduction of accessories and water channel for the irrigation of bile duct (**Figures 5** and **6**).

4.1 Stages of laparoscopic CBD manipulation by cholangioscope

4.1.1 Stage 1: Installation of patient

Our team uses the standard dorsal lithotomy position of patient on the table with abducted legs for laparoscopic approach. The surgeon stands between the legs of the patients with the camera man standing on the left of the patient and the first assistant on the patient's right. This is the same patient's operative position, which we also use for laparoscopic cholecystectomy.

4.1.2 Stage 2: Creation of pneumoperitoneum and trocars placement

During the procedure, we utilize a 30° optic camera with the monitor placed on the patient's right. Usually, pneumoperitoneum is created with a Veress needle by

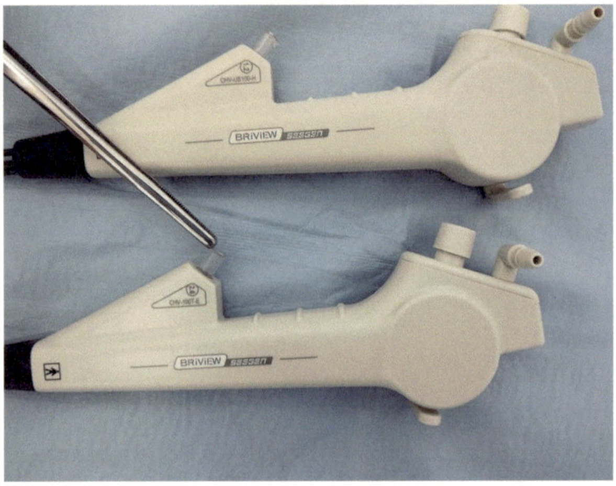

Figure 5.
Choledochoscope – working channel.

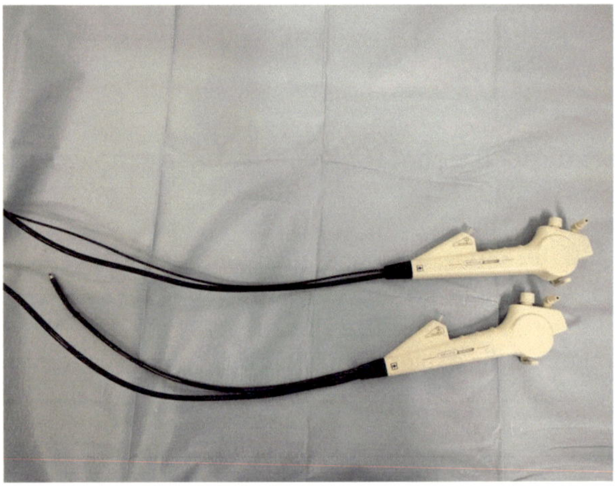

Figure 6.
Choledochoscope – 3 and 5 mm.

infra-umbilical or trans-umbilical approach creating pressure up to 12 mm Hg. If the patient has a previous laparotomy, we apply the open technique with the introduction of Hasson cannula. For the camera port, we use this first 10 mm trocar (T1). All the rest trocars are introduced under direct vision with the camera. The second 10 mm trocar (T2) is positioned at about 5–7 cm above the umbilicus along the midline and connected to gas supply hose avoiding a blurred vision of the camera. Two additional trocars of 5 mm are placed along the right anterior axillary line and right midclavicular line (T3 and T4) at the level of umbilicus. T3 is used by the first assistant to apply the fundus traction of gallbladder. T2 and T4 are working trocars for the surgeon. For distal exploration of common bile duct (CBD) with choledochoscope, we use 5 mm T5 trocar placed immediately below the right costal arch. For the proximal exploration of the CBD, we utilize the 5 mm T4 trocar if we apply 3 mm flexible choledochoscope for exploration. If we use the flexible 5 mm choledochoscope, we replace 5 mm T4 trocar with a larger 10 mm port (**Figure 7**).

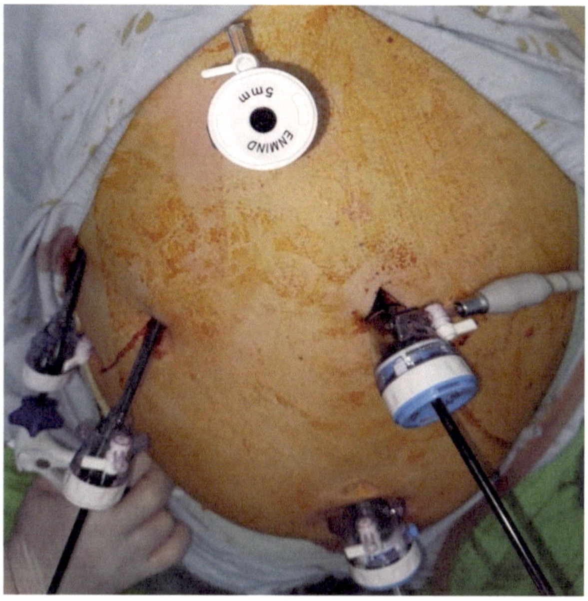

Figure 7.
Patient with lithotomy position on the table – trocar placement.

4.1.3 Stage 3: Dissection of hepatoduodenal ligament and CBD

The peritoneum overlying the CBD was divided by scissors, and we start dissection around the cystic duct and along the hepatoduodenal ligament through the use of bipolar electrocautery avoiding the current diffusion to the CBD and arteries. Dissection and separation of cystic duct, cystic artery, and CBD should be done with meticulous care. The cystic duct is clamped first and cut off at least 5–10 mm to the confluence, to avoid stone migration into the CBD during manupulation and to be long enough for trans-cystic approach. The cystic artery was also clamped and cut. We dissect and explore the anterior wall of the CBD with care to avoid the hemorrhage from venous and arterial paracholedochal plexuses. Usually, 10 mm dissection of the anterior surface of CBD would suffice to do choledochotomy.

After the dissection of the cystic duct and cystic artery and their division between the titanium clips, we keep the gallbladder in place attached to the liver. The first assistant applies cephalic traction on the fundus of the bladder by grasper to raise the liver and to expose the hepatoduodenal ligament and to help the dissection of its structures (**Figure 8**).

4.1.4 Stage 4: Choledochotomy and insertion of a cholangioscope

During the dissection of CBD, the second assistant sustaining traction on duodenum and first assistant keeping the traction on the gallbladder's fundus the surgeon place two stay sutures on each side of the bile duct. By applying traction on the stay sutures, we open with scissors the CBD through longitudinal choledochotomy over 1 cm (**Figure 9**).

We usually explore the CBD through the choledochotomy. Less frequently, our surgeon applies a transcystic approach. The choice depends on the size, number, position of stones in the bile duct, the diameter of cystic duct, and CBD.

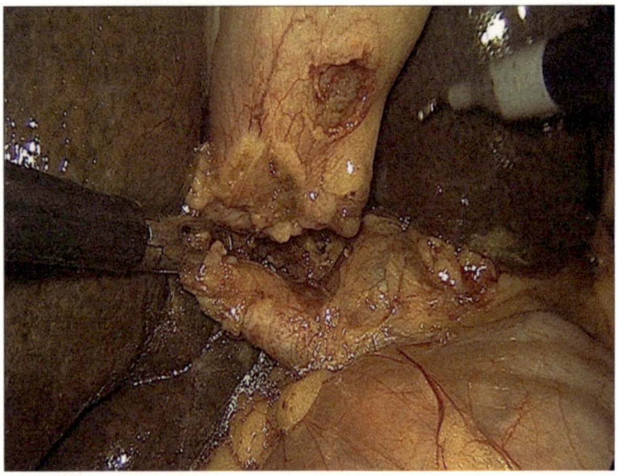

Figure 8.
Dissection of hepatoduodenal ligament.

We apply the following indications for the choledochotomy approach:

1. The diameter of CBD more than 10 mm.

2. Stones larger than CBD's diameter.

3. Number of stones ≥3.

4. Proximal position of stone in the CBD (above the confluence of cystic duct).

5. The diameter of cystic duct <4 mm.

Our choice to open the CBD is a longitudinal choledochotomy with scissors because we could remove larger stones by enlarging the incision and found no risk of long-term ischemic complications of the CBD (**Figure 10**). The choledochoscope can be introduced without difficulties into the biliary tract through this choledochotomy. Insertion of the device could be towards the duodenum (for distal exploration) or towards the liver (for proximal exploration).

4.1.5 Stage 5: Exploration of CBD by cholangioscope and stone extraction

The maneuvering of the choledochoscope in the bile duct could be very challenging (**Figure 11**). It depends on the surgeon's experience and the assistant's help. Usually, for distal exploration of bile duct, the surgeon introduces the choledochoscope through the T5 port. The scope is advanced under direct vision in the same manner as we navigate a rectoscope. The first assistant applies continuous traction on the duodenum by a soft fenestrated clamp to help the surgeon with choledochoscope's introduction into the CBD. The second surgeon takes control of the handle of a choledochoscope with saline's irrigation and visualization of the CBD. The tip of the choledochoscope is navigated inside the bile duct and down through the papilla to the duodenum to identify the ductal stones. If there is an obstruction of CBD, we apply different techniques for stone retrieval, adapting to each case. This could be a

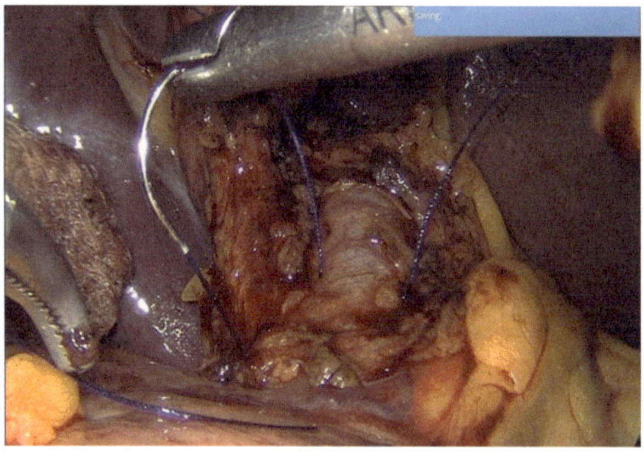

Figure 9.
Placement of stay suture on the CBD.

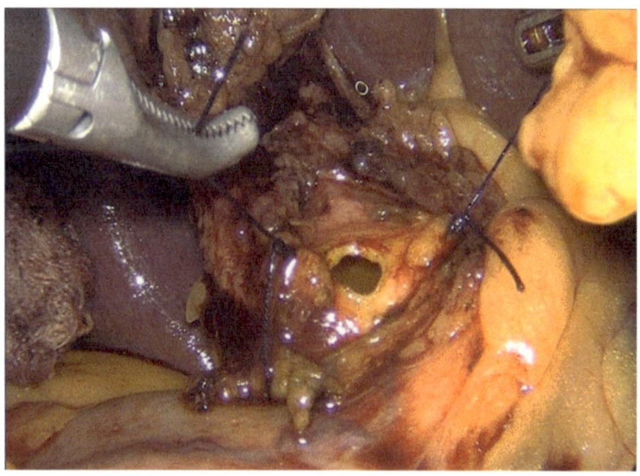

Figure 10.
Longitudinal choledochotomy – 10 mm length.

Dormia basket, an irrigation catheter, and a Fogarty balloon catheter. Positioning of the choledochoscope close to the stone in the CBD and advancement of the extraction catheter beyond the stone gives the chance for stone withdrawal with the choledochoscope (**Figures 12** and **13**).

We always repeat the choledochoscopy of the CBD after stone retrieval to check for retained stones. The surgeon confirms the permeability of the papilla reaching the duodenum (**Figure 14**). For us, this is a positive sign that there is no residual stone. We always explore the proximal bile duct through T4 port. For us, there is no need for intraoperative cholangiography at the end of examination (IOC) to confirm the absence of residual stones.

If there is no residual stone, we close the CBD with 4/0 polyglactin suture with placement of T-tube external biliary drainage.

Almost all the patients in our series are presenting clinical signs of papillary edema, cholangitis, or acute pancreatitis at the admission, needing extraction of multiple bile duct stones. The surgeon always checks the bile-proof around the T-tube by infusion of saline through the external drainage (**Figure 15**).

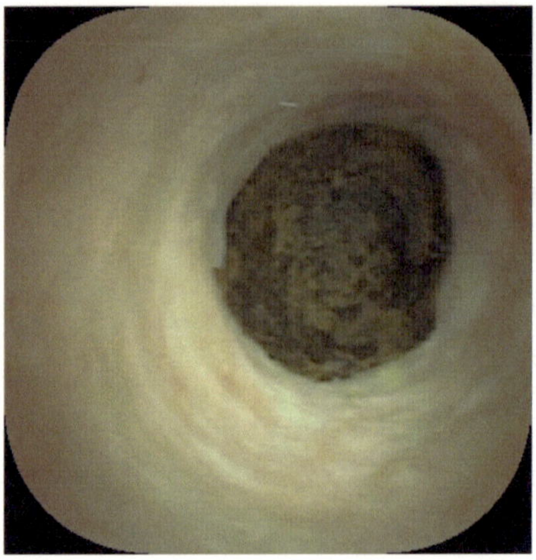

Figure 11.
Stone in the distal CBD.

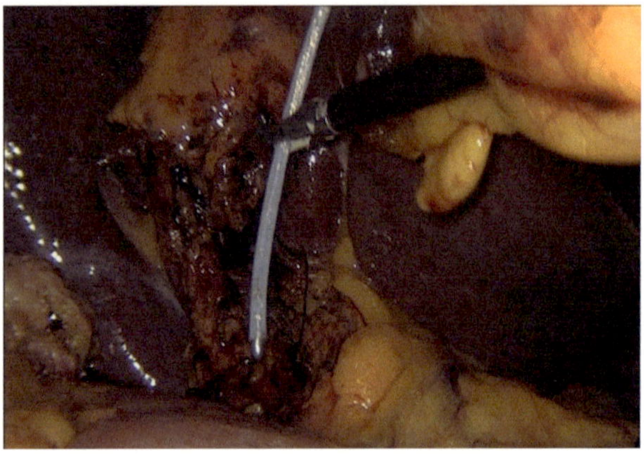

Figure 12.
Dormia basket in the distal BD.

We close the T-tube on the next day, and we do a transdrainage cholangiography on the 21st day. In the case of good visualization of intrahepatic bile ducts and duodenum and no residual stones, we remove the T-tube. During the follow-up period, we found no stenosis of the CBD and no postoperative bile leakage in our series.

After the closure of the CD around the T-tube, we put a subhepatic contact drain close to the hepatoduodenal ligament.

4.1.6 Stage 6: Completion of cholecystectomy

We complete the retrograde cholecystectomy, and the gallbladder is removed with a specimen retrieval bag.

4.1.7 Stage 7: Closure of ports opening

We close the opening of the abdominal wall with 2/0 Vicryl sutures after irrigation with povidone iodine solution and 0.25% 10 ml bupivacaine injection.

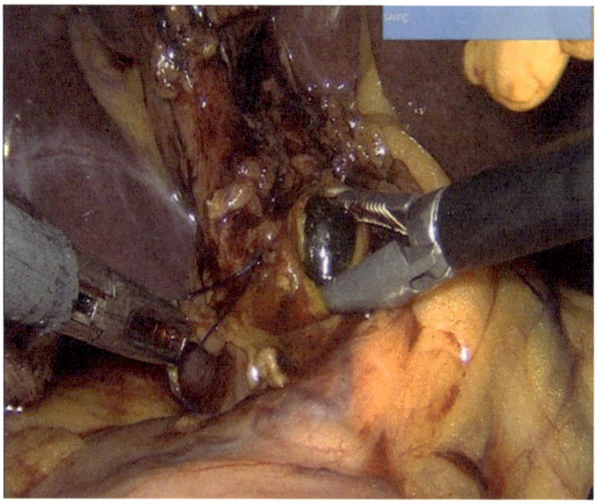

Figure 13.
Stone extraction from the distal CBD.

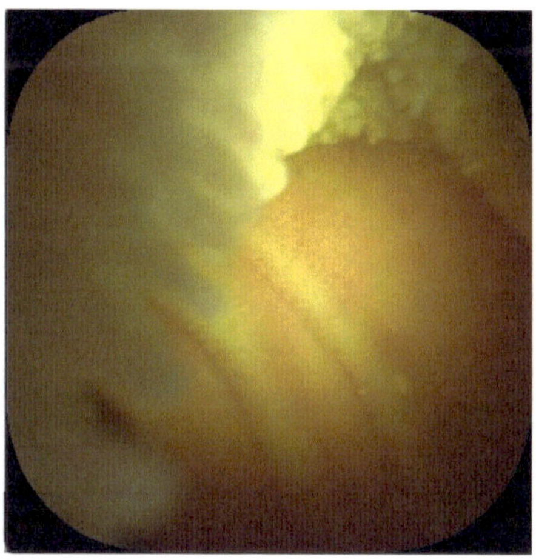

Figure 14.
Choledochoscope into the duodenum-confirms the permeability of the papilla—no residual stones.

In cases where the extraction of the stones was impossible through laparoscopic access, we perform laparotomy with an oblique mini-incision, usually 2 cm below the right costal margin. This skin incision is about 4–5 cm long. We do this intervention only for the exploration of the CBD by cholangioscope. Usually, the gallbladder is removed before that through laparoscopic approach. During the open operation again, we dissect the anterior wall of the CBD and place stay sutures 4/0 PDS on each site of the CBD. Applying traction on the stay sutures, we cut longitudinally the bile duct about 10 mm long. Introduction of the choledochoscope first distally and then in the opposite direction helps us to explore the inner surface of CBD. When the stones were found, they were extracted by Dormia basket, Fogarty catheter, or forceps. After verification by the cholangioscope (always passing through the papilla of Vateri) that there is no residual stone in the CBD, we place routinely 8-10Fr T-tube to decrease the pressure in the bile system and for postoperative cholangiography. We always fix the T-tube to the skin by multiple 5/0 nonabsorbable sutures.

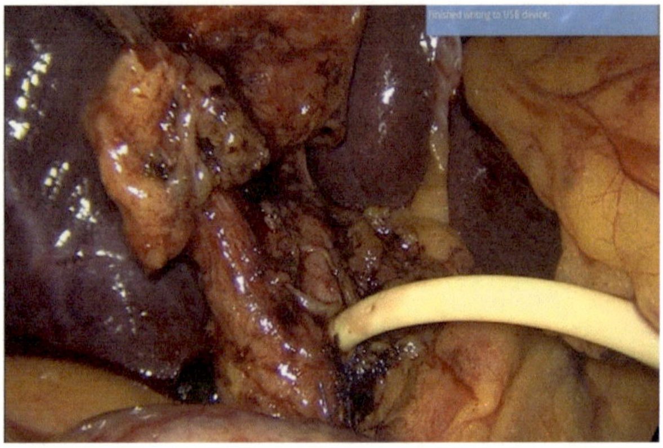

Figure 15.
Placement of T-tube into the CBD.

5. Discussion

In this study, we apply efficiently the laparoscopic approach for the CBDE by a cholangioscope. The patients were presenting signs of acute cholecystitis or complication of bile duct stones. In these complicated cases, dissection and insertion of the cholangioscope into the CBD may pose many technical problems and may increase the risk of intraoperative hemorrhage. We suggest that careful handling of tissue, cautious manipulation of choledochoscope into the bile duct, and the experience of surgeon could avoid these problems even in elderly patients with complicated cholecystolithiasis and choledocholithiasis.

For the exploration of choledoch, many authors prefer longitudinal choledochotomy over a distance of approximately 1 cm, but others prefer horizontal incision. The benefit of vertical incision is the possibility of enlargement in the case of bigger stones. The horizontal approach avoids ischemia of CBD. Usually, the surgeon uses 4-0 monofilament absorbable sutures for closure of the incision [33–36].

In our study, we prefer longitudinal incision of the CBD over 1 cm. This length is always enough to extract the stone. We do not use primary closure of choledoch. We speculate that ischemia of the CBD depends on the meticulous dissection around the choledoch and avoidance of vessel damage around the CBD. With our technique of choledochotomy, we have not seen stenosis of the CBD after operation.

After extraction of stones through the choledochotomy, there are two possibilities: closure of bile duct either primarily or over a T-tube. The indication for T-tube insertion is decompression of the duct in patients with cholangitis, residual distal obstruction without stones, or to confirm the absence of residual stones in the CBD by cholangiography in the postoperative period. Some centers use transcystic tubes or antegrade stenting of CBD. The advocates for primary closure explain this with avoidance of drainage dislodgement, bile leakage, and infection.

In our study, there was no bile leakage, no drain dislodgment, or bile peritonitis in the postoperative period. There was no patient with hemorrhage or infection complication. Our preference is a closure over 8Fr-10Fr T- tube. We suppose that decreasing pressure in the CBD is very important prerequisite to avoid complications in patients with acute cholecystitis, trauma of CBD after bile stone extraction. To avoid bile leakage and tube dislodgement, the surgeon always checks the bile-proof around the

T-tube by infusion of saline through the external drainage, and if there is a suspicion, he adds additional suture around the drainage tube. We always fix the T-tube to the skin with 5/0 nonabsorbable sutures.

From these 32 patients enrolled in our study, 21 patients are more than 75 years and presenting comorbidities in 22 cases. All the patients are admitted with acute cholecystitis with or without some complications of choledocholithiasis.

Our results confirm the report of Yong Yan et al. that the early one-stage operation (LCBDE+LC) for patients with acute cholecystitis and choledocholithiasis is acceptable with achieving clearance of CBD stones and low morbidity [32]. We also agree with the published meta-analysis including 693 elderly patients that LCBDE is a safe and effective treatment for elderly patients with choledocholithiasis. We cannot confirm the remarks of this study for higher pulmonary complications in these patients [37].

At the end, we also suggest that LCBDE is a safe and effective method, but there is a learning curve to accomplish these acceptable results. According to some studies, the authors conclude that the learning curve of LCBDE was achieved after the accomplishment of 54–60 cases [38, 39].

6. Conclusions

We found that the laparoscopic intraoperative cholangioscopy is a reliable diagnostic and therapeutic method for CBD stones. It is a reliable approach even in the cases of complicated forms of acute cholecystitis in elderly patients. Although not conventionally adopted, the laparoscopic intraoperative cholangioscopy is a safe, physiological, and efficient method in experienced hands.

Author details

Sotirov Dobromir Yordanov[1*] and Petar Filev[2]

1 MBAL “Sveti Panteleimon AD”, Yambol, Bulgaria

2 Saint Panteleimon's Hospital, Yambol, Bulgaria

*Address all correspondence to: sotirovdr@fastmail.com

References

[1] Ashby BS. Choledochoscopy. Clinics in Gastroenterology. 1978;7:685-700

[2] Courvoisier L. Casuistisch-Staiistische Beitraye zur Patholoyie und Chirurgie der Gallenwenge. Leipzig: Vogel; 1890: 28 & 1

[3] Babcock WW. Management of biliary diseases and their surgical complications. Penn Medicine Journal. 1937;**604**

[4] Hollenberg HG, Eikner WC. Cholecystoscopy. Surgery. 1937;**2**:37

[5] Mclver MA. Instrument for visualizing interior of the common duct at operation. Surgery. 1941;**9**:112

[6] Wildegans VH. Grenzen der Cholangiographie und Aussichten der Endoskopie der Tiefen Gallenwege. Med K/in 35. 1953;**35**:1270

[7] Freitas ML, Bell RL, Duffy AJ. Choledocholithiasis: Evolving standards for diagnosis and management. World Journal of Gastroenterology. 2006;**12**:3162-3167

[8] Shore JM, Shore E. Operative biliary endoscopy experience with the flexible choledochoscope in 100 consecutive choledocholithotomies. Annals of Surgery. 1970;**171**:269

[9] Shore JM, Morgenstern L, Berci G. An improved rigid choledochoscope. The American Journal of Surgery. 1971;**122**:567

[10] Mauro A, Mazza S, Scalvini D, et al. The role of cholangioscopy in biliary diseases. Diagnostics. 2023;**13**:2933. DOI: 10.3390/diagnostics13182933

[11] Xu S, Zhong G, Minghui D, Yu J, Wan G, Mingjun X. Comparison of the effect and cost of laparoscopy and laparotomy in the treatment of gallbladder complicated with common bile duct stones. Journal of Qingdao University (Medical Edition). 2020;**56**(1):76-79

[12] Shore JM, Manitoba MD, et al. A flexible choledochoscope. The Lancet. 1965;**285**(7397):1200-1201

[13] Kim HJ, Choi HS, Park JH, Park DI, Cho YK, Sohn CI, et al. Factors influencing the technical difficulty of endoscopic clearance of bile duct stones. Gastrointestinal Endoscopy. 2007;**66**:1154-1160

[14] Quaresima S, Balla A, Guerrieri M, et al. A 23 year experience with laparoscopic common bile duct exploration. HPB. 2017;**19**(1):29-35. DOI: 10.1016/j.hpb.2016.10.011. Epub 2016 Nov 24

[15] Dasari BV, Tan CJ, Gurusamy KS, Martin DJ, Kirk G, McKie L, et al. Surgical versus endoscopic treatment of bile duct stones. Cochrane Database of Systematic Reviews. 2013;**2013**:CD003327

[16] Sandha J, van Zanten SV, Sandha G. The safety and efficacy of single-operator cholangioscopy in the treatment of difficult common bile duct stones after failed conventional ERCP. Journal of the Canadian Association of Gastroenterology. 2018;**1**:181-190

[17] Pan L, Chen M, Ji L, Zheng L, Yan P, Fang J, et al. The safety and efficacy of laparoscopic common bile duct exploration combined with cholecystectomy for the management of cholecysto-choledocholithiasis: An

up-to-date meta-analysis. Annals of Surgery. 2018;**268**:247-253

[18] Van Dijk AH, Lamberts M, van Laarhoven CJ, et al. Laparoscopy in cholecysto-choledocholithiasis. Best Practice & Research. Clinical Gastroenterology. 2014;**28**:195-209

[19] Manes G, Paspatis G, Aabakken L, Anderloni A, Arvanitakis M, Ah-Soune P, et al. Endoscopic management of common bile duct stones: European Society of Gastrointestinal Endoscopy (ESGE) guideline. Endoscopy. 2019;**51**:472-491

[20] Ong TZ, Khor JL, Selamat DS, Yeoh KG, Ho KY. Complications of endoscopic retrograde cholangiography in the post-MRCP era: A tertiary center experience. World Journal of Gastroenterology. 2005;**11**:5209-5212

[21] Schreurs WH, Juttmann JR, Stuifbergen WN, Oostvogel HJ, van Vroonhoven TJ. Management of common bile duct stones: Selective endoscopic retrograde cholangiography and endoscopic sphincterotomy: Short- and long-term results. Surgical Endoscopy. 2002;**16**:1068-1072

[22] Shelat VG, Chia VJ, Low J. Common bile duct exploration in an elderly Asian population. International Surgery. 2015;**100**:261-267

[23] Po-Hsuan W, Min-Wei Y, et al. Comparison of laparoscopic common bile duct exploration plus cholecystectomy and endoscopic retrograde cholangiopancreatography followed by laparoscopic cholecystectomy for elderly patients with common bile duct stones and gallbladder stones. Journal of Gastrointestinal Surgery. 2024;**28**(5):719-724

[24] Kharbutli B, Velanovich V. Management of preoperatively suspected choledocholithiasis: A decision analysis. Journal of Gastrointestinal Surgery. 2008;**12**(11):1973-1980

[25] Al-Ardah M, Barnett RE, et al. Lessons learnt from the first 200 unselected consecutive cases of laparoscopic exploration of common bile duct stones at a district general hospital. Surgical Endoscopy. 2021;**35**(11):6268-6277

[26] Lan W-F, Li J-H, Wang Q-B, et al. Comparison of laparoscopic common bile duct exploration and endoscopic retrograde cholangiopancreatography combined with laparoscopic cholecystectomy for patients with gallbladder and common bile duct stones a meta-analysis of randomized controlled trials. European Review for Medical and Pharmacological Sciences. 2023;**27**:4656-4669

[27] Grubnik VV, Tkachenko AI, et al. Laparoscopic common bile duct versus open surgery: Comparative prospective randomized trial. Surgical Endoscopy. 2012;**26**:2165-2171

[28] Berthou JC, Dron B, et al. Evaluation of laparoscopic treatment of common bile duct stones in a prospective series of 505 patients: Indications and results. Surgical Endoscopy. 2007;**21**:1970-1974

[29] Aydin MC, Karahan SR, Kose E. Comparison between laparoscopic and conventional technique in the surgical treatment of choledocholithiasis. Laparoscopic Endoscopic Surgical Science. 2020;**27**(3):122-129

[30] Sharma A, Dahiya P, et al. Management of common bile duct stones in the laparoscopic era. The Indian Journal of Surgery. 2012;**74**:264-269

[31] Madhsoudi H, Garadaghi A, et al. Biliary peritonitis requiring reoperation

after removal of T-tubes from the common bile duct. American Journal of Surgery. 2005;**190**:430-433

[32] Yan Y, Sha Y, et al. One-stage versus two-stage management for acute cholecystitis associated with common bile duct stones: A retrospective cohort study. Surgical Endoscopy. 2022;**36**(2):920-929

[33] Petelin JB. Laparoscopic common bile duct exploration. Surgical Endoscopy. 2003;**17**(11):1705-1715

[34] Isla AM, Griniatsos J, Karvounis E, Arbuckle JD. Advantages of laparoscopic stented choledochorrhaphy over T-tube placement. British Journal of Surgery. 2004;**91**(7):862-866

[35] Hotta T, Taniguchi K, Kobayashi Y, et al. Biliary drainage tube evaluation after common bile duct exploration for choledocholithiasis. Hepato-Gastroenterology. 2003;**50**(50):315-321

[36] Kitano S, Bandoh T, Yoshida T, Shuto K. Laparoscopic C-tube drainage via cystic duct following common bile duct exploration. Journal of Hepato-Biliary-Pancreatic Surgery. 1995;**2**(2):146-149

[37] Zhu J, Shuju T, Yang Z, et al. Laparoscopic common bile duct exploration for elderly patients with choledocholithiasis: A systematic review and meta-analysis. Surgical Endoscopy. 2020;**34**(4):1522-1533

[38] Duran M, Silvestre J, Hernández J, et al. Learning curve for performing laparoscopic common bile duct exploration in biliary surgery 2.0 era. Journal of Hepato-Biliary-Pancreatic Sciences. 2023;**30**(3):374-382

[39] Zhu H, Linquan W, Yuan R, et al. Learning curve for performing choledochotomy bile duct exploration with primary closure after laparoscopic cholecystectomy. Surgical Endoscopy. 2018;**32**(10):4263-4270

Chapter 5

Emerging Techniques in Management of Biliary Tract Diseases

Sree Harshitha Vallabhaneni,
Sri Sravya Lalitha Chandrika Thungathurthi,
Prem Kurra and Supraj Teeparthy

Abstract

In this book chapter, we discuss emerging techniques in three important aspects of biliary tract diseases: diagnostic, pharmacological, and procedural advancements. We begin the chapter by highlighting the importance and need for advancements in improving the quality of life in patients. We examined the latest advancements in diagnostic technologies that facilitate early disease detection, including the identification of biomarkers and molecular markers in serum and bile. We also delve into the use of liquid biopsies, genetic testing and innovations in magnetic resonance cholangiopancreatography (MRCP). In light of the increasing role of artificial intelligence, we discuss how AI is being leveraged to enhance diagnostic accuracy. In the subsequent section, we highlight advances in pharmacological management and address procedural advancements in techniques for stone removal and stenting, including Endoscopic Retrograde Cholangiopancreatography (ERCP). We explore cholangioscopic methods, such as direct visualisation techniques. This section also explores advancements in Percutaneous Transhepatic Cholangiography (PTC) and several ablation methods for treating biliary tumours. Furthermore, it addresses the enhancements in minimally invasive procedures, such as laparoscopic surgery. Robotic systems are increasingly pivotal in enhancing precision across various medical disciplines. Additionally, we discuss emerging modalities such as gene therapy and regenerative medicine, highlighting their growing prominence. The potential of gene therapy to correct genetic disorders affecting the biliary tract and the use of stem cell therapy for repairing biliary damage and regenerating bile ducts in autoimmune diseases are examined. We conclude the chapter by emphasising the importance of integrating advanced and traditional techniques to provide optimal patient care and enhance quality of life.

Keywords: innovation, diagnostic, pharmacological, biliary tract diseases, advancement

1. Introduction

Biliary tract diseases include a wide spectrum of diseases including congenital anomalies (Choledochal Cyst, Choledocholithiasis), Inflammatory conditions (Suppurative Cholangitis, Primary Sclerosing Cholangitis, Recurrent Pyogenic Cholangitis, IgG4-Related Cholangitis), Neoplasms of the biliary tract (Benign Tumours of the Bile Ducts like *Biliary Hamartoma, Biliary Cystadenoma, Intraductal Papillary Neoplasm of the Bile Duct (IPNB);* Malignant Tumours of the Bile Ducts), Functional biliary disorders(biliary dyskinesia) and Diseases of the gallbladder (Including cholecystitis, cholelithiasis and gallbladder cancer) [1].

There are a variety of risk factors that increase the chance of biliary tract diseases. A majority of these factors have a history of chronic biliary epithelial damage and long-term inflammation [2].

Risk factors for biliary tract cancer include several lifestyle and biological factors such as smoking, gallstones, parasitic or bacterial infections of the biliary tract, hypercholesterolemia, high caloric and carbohydrate diets, female gender, age, cigarette smoking, alcohol intake, excess body weight, postmenopausal status in women, and history of cholecystectomy or hysterectomy [2, 3]. Additional risks include inflammatory bowel disease, diabetes, and consumption of sucrose and sweetened beverages. Numerous pathogens have also been implicated, including mycotoxins, Salmonella Typhi/Paratyphi, Helicobacter bilis/pylori, and hepatitis B and C viruses. Other suspected risk factors for biliary tract cancer, such as reproductive factors and obesity, probably alter the risk of biliary tract cancer by increasing or decreasing the risk of gallstones [2]. The mechanism linking gallstones and biliary tract cancer is still unknown, but it may be related to infection or irritation caused by the stones [2].

Some countries, such as Japan, Poland, various South American countries, and certain racial groups (Native American Indians) have excessively high rates for biliary tract cancer might also be explained by a high frequency of lithogenic genes. Tumours of the bilio-pancreatic organs are much more frequent than those arising from the small bowel and are much more aggressive. Within the biliary tract, tumours of the gallbladder are more frequent than tumours of the ductal system [2].

Several recent studies have suggested that, globally, biliary tract cancer (BTC) incidence and mortality rates have been increasing in recent decades, with intrahepatic cholangiocarcinoma (ICC) showing an average annual rise of 4.36% [4]. While mortality rates are generally decreasing in many countries, regions like Chile, Greece, the UK, and Germany have seen significant increases, particularly among women [5].

Therefore, bringing about a need for a higher degree of diagnostic accuracy that can detect biliary tract diseases early at their onset or their risk factors (gallstones, infections, gallbladder polyps, and other inflammatory conditions) and treatment modalities that can hit hard and hit fast.

In this chapter, we will explore the diagnostic, pharmacological, and procedural advancements that make sense this possible, including targeted therapies, Percutaneous Trans-Hepatic Cholangiography (PTC), MRCP, DWI, CEUS and other non-invasive modalities.

The ongoing innovations in MRCP and other non-invasive imaging modalities are transforming the landscape of biliary tract disease diagnosis and management. With the advent of 3D imaging, enhanced contrast techniques, diffusion-weighted imaging, novel radiotracers, and AI-driven analysis, clinicians are better equipped than ever to diagnose biliary pathologies with precision and guide treatment decisions.

2. Imaging and diagnostic innovations

2.1 Advanced imaging techniques

Accurate characterisation and staging of the malignancies, made possible with multimodality imaging, will determine respectability and impact on subsequent management [6].

In recent years, advancements in imaging technology have significantly improved the diagnosis and management of biliary tract diseases. Magnetic Resonance Cholangiopancreatography (MRCP) has emerged as a leading non-invasive modality, offering clinicians a high-resolution, contrast-free method for evaluating biliary and pancreatic ducts. Alongside MRCP, other innovative imaging techniques such as contrast-enhanced ultrasound (CEUS), diffusion-weighted imaging (DWI), and novel radiotracers in PET/CT have further refined diagnostic capabilities [6].

2.1.1 Magnetic resonance cholangiopancreatography (MRCP)

MRCP is a specialised MRI sequence that allows for the detailed visualisation of the biliary and pancreatic ductal systems. It leverages heavily T2-weighted MRI sequences, which are highly sensitive to static or slow-moving fluids like bile. By enhancing the signal from these fluids while suppressing signals from surrounding non-fluid tissues, MRCP generates high-contrast images that delineate the ductal structures. This allows for detailed visualisation of the biliary and pancreatic systems without the need for intravenous contrast agents, making it particularly useful in diagnosing obstructions, strictures, or other pathologies in these areas [7]. Recent innovations in MRCP technology have further enhanced its diagnostic utility:

- 3D MRCP: Three-dimensional MRCP offers a detailed, accurate view of biliary anatomy, achieving 100% sensitivity for typical structures and effectively assessing complex bifurcations and ductal variations. The improved spatial resolution facilitates the identification of subtle strictures, stones, or masses [8].

- MRCP with secretin stimulation: The administration of secretin, a hormone that stimulates the secretion of bile and pancreatic juices, enhances the visualisation of the pancreatic ducts and can help diagnose subtle obstructions or ductal anomalies that might be missed on standard MRCP sequences. The use of secretin with MRCP allows for dynamic evaluation of pancreatic exocrine function, which standard MRCP cannot achieve. However, the added costs, extended examination time, and the need for a nurse to administer the IV infusion have limited its widespread adoption in radiology practices [7].

- MRCP with diffusion-weighted imaging (DWI): DWI assesses water molecule movement within tissues, helping differentiate between benign and malignant biliary strictures, as malignant tissues typically restrict water movement more than benign ones. Combining MRCP with DWI improves the characterisation of biliary lesions, including cholangiocarcinoma [9].

2.1.2 Contrast-enhanced ultrasound (CEUS)

CEUS is an ultrasound technique that uses microbubble contrast agents to enhance the visualisation of the vascularisation of tissues. CEUS distinguishes benign from malignant biliary lesions by providing real-time imaging of bile ducts and characterising pathologies like gallbladder carcinoma by evaluating enhancement patterns, offering a non-invasive alternative to biopsy [10].

2.1.3 Diffusion-weighted imaging (DWI)

DWI is increasingly being used in conjunction with MRCP to enhance the diagnostic accuracy of biliary tract disease assessment. By evaluating the movement of water molecules in tissues, DWI can identify areas of abnormal cellular density, a hallmark of malignant transformation [11]. Innovations in DWI include:

- Improved characterisation of cholangiocarcinoma: DWI has shown potential in differentiating cholangiocarcinoma from benign biliary strictures, as malignant lesions typically exhibit restricted diffusion. This can aid in the early detection and accurate staging of cholangiocarcinoma, which is crucial for planning therapeutic interventions [11].

- Assessment of post-surgical complications: DWI can help identify post-operative complications such as biliary leaks or abscesses by highlighting areas of abnormal fluid accumulation, providing valuable information that can guide management decisions [11].

2.1.4 Positron emission tomography (PET/CT) with novel radiotracers

PET/CT imaging has gained traction in the evaluation of biliary tract diseases, particularly in the context of cancer diagnosis and staging. The development of novel radiotracers that target specific metabolic pathways has improved the sensitivity and specificity of PET/CT in detecting biliary malignancies. F-18 FDG PET/CT is particularly effective in localising and staging cholangiocarcinoma, while emerging tracers like Ga-68 DOTATATE enhance the diagnosis of neuroendocrine tumours by targeting specific receptors, enabling more accurate and tailored treatment [12].

2.1.5 Elastography

Ultrasound elastography (UE) measures tissue elasticity using an ultrasound probe. Elastography is a non-invasive technique that assesses tissue stiffness, essential for diagnosing biliary diseases. It includes strain imaging, which uses external or internal forces, and shear wave imaging, which employs dynamic stress. Shear wave imaging features Transient Elastography (TE) for liver stiffness and real-time assessment to distinguish between benign and malignant biliary strictures [13].

2.1.6 Artificial intelligence (AI) in imaging

The integration of artificial intelligence (AI) into biliary tract imaging is one of the most exciting recent developments. AI algorithms are being developed to assist in the interpretation of imaging studies, potentially improving diagnostic accuracy and reducing human error. Key innovations include:

- AI in MRCP interpretation: AI-driven software aids radiologists by automatically identifying and characterising biliary lesions, streamlining diagnosis, and predicting treatment response and disease progression. It helps forecast complications in chronic conditions like PSC, enabling earlier intervention [14].

That said, there are several disadvantages to using AI in clinical settings: algorithms often perform poorly with real-world data, can introduce bias, and may have opaque decision-making processes. Additionally, managing AI costs, ensuring clear accountability, and addressing ethical concerns are critical for successful implementation [15].

2.2 Biomarkers and molecular diagnostics

Tumour markers can be used for tumour screening, early detection, differential diagnosis and staging, prognosis judgement, efficacy monitoring, recurrence and metastasis monitoring, and guiding individualised treatment [16].

An ideal tumour marker:

- Simple and affordable (widely available).
- Highly sensitive (to detect the disease at an early stage, preferably when curative therapy can be provided), and specific (to distinguish Biliary tract cancer from other malignant or benign diseases).
- Reflect the tumour's dynamic changes [16].
- The detection of tumour markers should be simple, fast, and accurate [16].

Advanced methods for measuring gene expression, proteins, and metabolites in body fluids and tissues are now accessible. These methods, known as "omics" technologies, aim to identify markers that can help understand tumour biology and identify new targets for treatment [17]. They can also help classify different clinical conditions, assess disease severity, and predict long-term outcomes for patients. "Omics" techniques include genomics for circulating tumour cells (CTCs) escaping from primary sites, extracellular vesicles (EV) containing nucleic acids and proteins, cell-free DNA and RNA released from tumour cells (including messenger RNA (mRNA), ribosomal RNA (RNA), and other noncoding RNA such as microRNAs (miRNA)), and proteins and metabolites secreted by tumour cells. These biomarkers offer additional opportunities for detecting and understanding cancer through non-invasive blood tests [17].

While the field of liquid biopsy (a method of diagnosing cancer by analysing blood samples) is still in its infancy, it has great potential for future developments.

Bile has complex components and is in direct contact with biliary tract tumours. Bile is composed mainly of bile acids, phospholipids, cholesterol, bilirubin, proteins, inorganic salts, etc. Proteins account for about 7% of the total bile composition (183). Under the condition of disease, the ingredients of bile can be changed, especially in terms of BTCs, which are directly in touch with bile [16]. Therefore, compared with blood or other body fluids, bile is an essential source for searching for tumour markers in the biliary system (**Table 1**) [16].

Biomarker type	**Biofluid**	**Biomarker**	
		Diagnostic biomarkers	**Prognostic biomarkers**
Genetic Biomarkers	Bile	1. ARID1A (AT-rich interaction domain 1A) 2. BAP1 (BRCA1-associated protein 1) 3. SMAD4 (SMAD family member 4)	• ARID1A, BAP1, SMAD4
	Blood	• CTNNB1 (catenin beta 1) • FGFR2 (fibroblast growth factor receptor 2) • IDH1/2 (isocitrate dehydrogenase 1 and 2) • PIK3CA (phosphatidylinositol 3-kinase) • TP53 (tumor protein p53) • KRAS (Kirsten rat sarcoma viral oncogene homolog) • BRAF (v-Raf murine sarcoma viral oncogene homolog B)	
	Serum	CTNNB1,FGFR2 , IDH1/2, PIK3CA , TP53 , KRAS , BRAF, SMAD4 (SMAD family member 4)	CTNNB1,FGFR2 , IDH1/2, PIK3CA , TP53 , KRAS , BRAF, SMAD4
Epigenetic Factors	**Blood**	• **HDAC6** (histone deacetylase 6) • **KMT2C** (lysine methyltransferase 2C) • **PBRM1** (polybromo 1) • **PTPN3** (protein tyrosine phosphatase non-receptor type 3) • **TGFß** (transforming growth factor beta)	
Transcriptomic biomarkers	Bile	**miR-9,miR-145,miR-105 , miR-147b,miR-302, miR-199-3p** : Are notable for their high sensitivity and specificity in distinguishing CCA and gallbladder carcinoma (GBC) from choledocholithiasis.	**miR-222**
	Serum	**miR-21, miR-26a**,miR-150,**miR-106a**,: Provides useful diagnostic information for identifying CCA **miR-126, miR**-1281,**miR-222**: Useful for distinguishing CCA from primary sclerosing cholangitis (PSC).	**miR-26a**: Besides its diagnostic value, it has potential for prognostic use in CCA
	Urine	miR-21 and miR-192 are potential biomarkers for O. viverrini-associated CCA	miR-21
Proteomic	Bile	SSP411 (Peptide Pattern)	
Metabolomic	Bile	Phosphatidylcholine, Bile Acids	
	Serum	**21-Deoxycortisol**: Used to assess adrenal function, which can be relevant in the context of biliary tract diseases if there is a suspicion of related adrenal involvement. **Bilirubin**: Key diagnostic marker for liver function and biliary obstruction, indicating conditions like cholestasis or biliary tract obstruction.	**LysoPC(14:0)**: Can be used to diagnose metabolic disturbances or liver dysfunctions associated with biliary tract diseases. **LysoPC(15:0)**: useful in diagnosing and potentially evaluating the severity of biliary tract diseases.

Table 1.
Biomarkers for biliary tract diseases [16–20].

3. Pharmacological advancements

3.1 Targeted therapy

Targeted therapy is one of the most innovative and newly emerging treatments. modalities that have changed the approach to cancer care. This approach focuses on attacking the root cause of the disease. It attacks specific mutated genes like fibroblast growth factor receptor (FGFR) gene, dehydrogenase isocitrate (IDH)-1 and 2, the BRAF protein-encoding gene (BRAF), breast cancer genes (BRCA1/2), epidermal growth factor receptor 2 (HER2), anaplastic lymphoma tyrosine kinase receptor (ALK), receptor tyrosine kinase-encoding proto-oncogene (RET), and neurotrophic receptor tyrosine kinase gene (NTRK).

Drugs targeting the FGFR gene, IDH 1 and 2 genes are most commonly being used in the treatment of intrahepatic cholangiocarcinomas (**Table 2**) [20].

3.2 Antibiotics

Antibiotics are widely used in infectious diseases of the biliary tract, like acute cholecystitis and cholangitis. Alongside general treatment methods like fluids and electrolyte correction, empirical therapy mostly directed towards enterobacteriaceae, specifically *E. Coli* is also being used. Drugs like ureidopenicillin, mezlocillin, piperacillin, or a combination of ampicillin plus aminoglycoside are widely used in the treatment of moderately severe cases of acute cholecystitis and cholangitis. Anaerobic cover for Bacteroides spp. is necessary in elderly patients, in patients with previous bile duct-bowel anastomosis, and with serious conditions. Recurrent cholangitis is being treated with agents like cotrimoxazole [21]. Recent researche has proven that prophylactic usage of Ertapenem (a new carbapenem antibiotic), Piperacillin, cefazolin, cefuroxime, cefotaxime, and ciprofloxacin is beneficial to avoid sepsis in patients with obstructive jaundice undergoing ERCP [21, 22].

S.no:	Target receptors	Examples of drugs
1	FGFR	Infigratinib, Erdafitinib, Pemigatinib, Derazantinib, futibatinib.
2	IDH 1	Ivosidenib
3	IDH2	Enasidenib
4	BRAF	Dabrafenib plus trametinib
5	BRCA 1/2	olaparib [Lynparza], rucaparib [Rubraca], niraparib [Zejula], and talazoparib [Talzenna]
6	HER2	Pertuzumab and trastuzumab Neratinib
7	ALK	Crizotinib (Xalkori),ceritinib (Zykadia),alectinib (Alecensa),brigatinib (Alunbrig),lorlatinib (Lorbrena)
8	RET	lenvatinib, sorafenib, alectinib, and sunitinib
9	NTRK	Entrectinib, Larotrectinib

Table 2.
Target receptors and the drugs that target them [20].

3.3 Pain management

About 20% of the adults develop gallstones, and the incidence is even more in the female population [23]. The most prominent symptom of cholelithiasis is pain. Pain due to gallstones is referred to as biliary colic. The mainstay of treatment for this symptom remains NSAIDs (non-steroidal anti-inflammatory drugs), diclofenac, ketorolac, tenoxicam, flurbiprofen, etc. [24]. Other than biliary colic, analgesic use is also very crucial in the postop phase of patient care. Anaesthetic drugs like lidocaine, ropivacaine, ketamine, bupivacaine, chloroprocaine, etc., are being used in various new routes like intraperitoneal instillation, nebulisation, central neuraxial blocks, transversus abdominis plane block, incisional infiltration, etc. [25]. Although each route has its own setbacks, it is proven that active pain management can speed up the recovery process and shorten hospital stay.

Apart from NSAIDs and anaesthetics, opioid drugs are also being used in severe acute and chronic pain. Drugs like Morphine, Fentanyl, Pethidine (meperidine), Buprenorphine, and Piritramide are being used. Due to their adverse effect, mainly addiction, newer drugs like Gabapentinoids (gabapentin, pregabalin, phenibut, etc.) are being used. Traditionally, these are used for neuropathic pain, but it is being said that usage of these drugs can reduce immediate postop pain and reduce the requirement of opioids in later stages [25].

3.4 Pharmacological treatment of autoimmune disorders

Primary biliary cholangitis is 10 times more common in women around 55 years of age than in men, whereas Primary sclerosing cholangitis is more common in men aged 30–40 years [26].

Ursodeoxycholic acid (UDCA) is the primary drug of choice for PBC. It is noted to have very minimal side effects, and a dose of 13–15 mg/kg/day is optimal [27]. In PBC non-reactive to UDCA, the use of fibrates like fenofibrate and bezafibrate can reduce alkaline phosphatase (ALP) levels and prevent liver cirrhosis [28]. Obeticholic acid (OCA), a semi-synthetic hydrophobic bile acid analogue, is also one of the licenced drugs that can be used for PBC. OCA has major limitations due to its side effects, like increased pruritus, leading to treatment non-adherence and derangement of lipid profiles. Budesonide can be added to UDCA in order to improve the liver's structure and function, whereas the proper efficacy of this treatment is still being researched. Fibrates can also be used with UDCA as an anti-cholestatic agent, but its safety is still a concern as it is shown to have some hepatotoxic effects. Full research on this treatment method is also awaited [27].

Although surgical therapy is the mainstay of treatment for PSC, new trials are being conducted on various pharmacological methods to give better patient care. Usage of bile acid modulator drugs like UDCA, OCA, non-bile acid farnesoid X receptor (FXR) agonists (Cilofexor), All-Trans retinoic acid plus UDCA, *nor*-UDCA are being studied; the results so far have been promising [29].

The use of fibrates like bezafibrate alongside UDCA has been a promising method to reduce fibrosis markers. It has been observed that MCP-1 expression is increased in cholangiocytes and livers of patients with PSC. Cenicriviroc is a dual antagonist of CCR2 and CCR5, which are the receptors for MCP-1. Usage of this also causes a reduction in inflammation. Timolumab is a monoclonal VAP-1 antibody, which reduces the entry of leukocytes. Vidolizumab is another new immunomodulator that targets the pathophysiology of PSC. Aldafermin acts on FGF19, which is related to limiting bile acid synthesis. Since bile acids are increased in PSC, this is also one of the treatment options, however, this drug is suspected to be carcinogenic. Simtuzumab acts by reducing the progression of fibrosis. Newer modalities like the ones mentioned in this section are constantly being researched. Although some of them have certain side effects, a few also have good potential to be used alongside surgical therapy in treating PSC. Other than bile and immunomodulators, microbiome manipulation using antibiotics and faecal transplant is also being studied [29].

4. Endoscopic advancements

4.1 Endoscopic retrograde cholangiopancreatography

ERCP is an endoscopic technique where a specially designed side-view endoscope is used to view the biliary and pancreatic ducts. The endoscope is designed in a way that the instruments needed to treat can also be sent in. ERCP is the mainstay diagnostic and therapeutic method for biliary strictures. Along with the endoscope, ultrasound is also used for accurate diagnosis. Biliary strictures can be either benign or malignant. Malignant strictures may be caused by cholangiocarcinoma or pancreatic adenocarcinoma. Understanding the aetiology is crucial for the effective treatment of biliary strictures. Obtaining a biopsy sample is made feasible with the help of ERCP. Therefore, ERCP serves as a valuable diagnostic tool for identifying these tumours. ERCP can also be used as a treatment modality for balloon dilation and stent placement and removal of gallstones. The transpapillary drainage technique can be used for drainage in acute cholecystitis in case the percutaneous approach is contraindicated. In patients with an inaccessible biliary tract, techniques like balloon enteroscope-assisted ERCP, Laparoscopic-assisted ERCP (LA-ERCP), or endoscopic ultrasound-directed transgastric ERCP (EDGE) are found to be extremely efficient. Novel techniques like ERCP-radiofrequency ablation are being used in the treatment of cancerous lesions [30].

4.2 New tools and techniques for stone removal

Spilled stones in the peritoneum can cause various complications like adhesions, fibrosis, abscess, etc. A new method of removal of these stones using laparoscopic graspers is being used. Small stones can be removed quickly using this method. Larger stones are broken into smaller pieces and removed [31].

A very promising non-surgical technique that has recently been developed is the use of extracorporeal shockwave lithotripsy (ESWL) for the treatment of gallbladder and biliary stones. This technique was previously used in the department of urology for renal stone removal. The usage of ESWL has reduced the need for general anaesthesia for stone removal. Using the piezoelectric technique has made it painless. Although this method has several short-term advantages, its effectiveness in the long run is still being studied. This method has a few limitations due to its uncertainty when it comes to the recurrence of the stone. To avoid recurrence, this method has to be followed by an adjuvant therapy using methyl-tert-butyl-ether (MTBE). Other than this, ESWL has also shown lung tissue damage and the development of arrhythmias in animal studies. Even though this method is very promising for the treatment of stones, the complications with this are yet to be dealt with [32].

4.3 New advancements in stents

Most preliminary inventions in this technique were self-expanding metal stents; however, the biliary tract, due to its extent, had a very high possibility of restenosis. To conquer this complication, the stents nowadays are being coated with various drugs [33]. A few examples of these coatings are:

4.3.1 Anticorrosive

Biodegradable stents are made with magnesium alloys. These alloys post degradation also act as anti-inflammatory and anticancer agents. However, this quick degradation process limits its effectiveness for clinical use. Hence anticorrosive coating has been added to tackle this complication. Coating the stents with polycaprolactone (PCL) and (JDBM) has significantly slowed down the corrosion. Nevertheless, this has been demonstrated in an *in vitro* environment, where the biliary tract's circumstances differ slightly. Thus, its effectiveness has not been established yet [33].

4.3.2 Antibacterial

One of the major risk factors of stenting is infection of the biliary tract. Biofilms can be formed on foreign bodies, leading to the formation of biliary sludge. Silver nanoparticles have been proven to be antiviral, anti-inflammatory, and antioxidants; hence, when used as a coating, they reduce the growth of organisms like *E. coli*, *Pseudomonas, Enterococcus*, and *Staphylococcus aureus*. In theory, an antibiotic coating on the stents would have an antibacterial effect; however, in experiments conducted on animals, neither antibiotic showed any advantages [33].

4.3.3 Antitumor

Antitumor coating has expanded the usage of stents beyond creating patency of the tracts. Antitumor coating is a great approach to treat biliary epithelial overgrowth and inward tumour cell expansion over the stent mesh through targeted therapy. Paclitaxel-drug-eluting stents and Gemcitabine-eluting stents have been proven to be most effective. That said, this technique, like every other, has its own limitations. These drugs can cause hypersecretion of mucin, bile duct epithelial separation, apart from their obvious effects on normal cells. All of these factors make it mandatory to weigh the risk-to-benefit ratio before using them [33].

4.3.4 Stone dissolving stents

Usage of sodium cholate (SC) can dissolve cholesterol stones, and ethylenediaminetetraacetic acid (EDTA) can dissolve pigment stones. These drugs have been proven to be significantly beneficial in both *in vitro* and animal studies. However, the uneven distribution of the drug poses a challenge. Hence, further studies are required to prove its safety for clinical use [33].

Other coatings being investigated include functional composite coatings, anti-stent migration coatings, and x-ray visible coatings. These new stent developments have a significant chance of becoming first-line therapeutic options in the future.

4.4 Innovations in managing ERCP-related complications

Major complications with ERCP are infections, post-ERCP pancreatitis, cholangitis, perforation and haemorrhage.

ERCP-related infection can be tackled with the use of preprocedural antibiotics. This method has been in practice for a long time, but nowadays post-procedural antibiotics for 3–5 days are also being used in special cases like post liver transplant strictures and patients with sclerosing cholangitis. Prompt percutaneous drainage, endoscopic decompression, and nasobiliary drainage procedures are being used in addition to the use of antibiotics and stents to guarantee appropriate post-operative drainage [34].

Post-ERCP pancreatitis most often leads to pancreatic necrosis. Necrosectomy was previously carried out with open surgery, but now it has been proven that percutaneous and laparoscopic methods have been more beneficial [34].

Post-ERCP cholangitis can be significantly reduced by reducing the usage of contrast for visualisation of the tract. Usage of methods like passing a guide wire and air cholangiography have been proven beneficial [34].

Post-ERCP haemorrhage can be tackled with balloon tamponade, injection of dilute epinephrine solution through a sclerotherapy needle, heater probe, or bipolar coagulation, and/or the placement of endoscopic clips. The most widely recognised and effective treatment for post-operative bleeding is epinephrine injection. Insertion of fully covered self-expandable metal stents (SEMS) into the bile duct is the newest method being used to treat bleeding refractory to traditional methods [34].

Another most dreaded complication of ERCP is perforation. Retroperitoneal perforation can be treated medically, whereas free intraperitoneal perforation requires immediate surgical repair.

4.5 Cholangioscopy

4.5.1 History and evolution

Cholangioscopy previously required two operators, presenting a significant challenge. Single operator cholangioscopy has been a frequently utilised diagnostic and therapeutic tool since its development.

4.5.2 Technique & visualization

Cholangioscopy is a type of direct visualisation technique that provides macroscopic analysis of the biliary mucosa. It can also be used as an addon to ER-US and ER-FNA for biopsy in case of malignant biliary strictures.

4.5.3 Access routes

Cholangioscopy was initially performed *via* the oral route; however, nowadays other routes like percutaneous, Trans-Cystic, Trans-Hepaticogastrostomy, and transpapillary have been explored [35].

4.5.4 Clinical indications

Usage of cholangioscopy has become crucial in the treatment of:

4.5.5 Indeterminate biliary strictures

If ERCP fails, cholangioscopy is the next best option for the diagnosis of biliary strictures. Cholangioscopy provides direct visualisation of the stricture as well as the surrounding mucosa. Malignancies are associated with surrounding neovascularisation, ulcer formation, and several other changes; all of these can be visualised through cholangioscopy. It has also been proven that cholangioscopy has fewer complications in comparison to endoscopic techniques [35].

4.5.6 Difficult gallstones

Cholangioscopy is also recently being used to treat gallstones using the lithotripsy technique. Electrohydraulic or laser energy is used to treat the stones. The usage of mechanical lithotripsy or endoscopic methods can be challenging to visualise the complete removal of the stones. Complete removal of the stones is mandatory to reduce post op complications. Therefore, peroral cholangioscopy is being used to visualise the biliary tract after the procedure.

4.5.7 Other applications

Cholangioscopy these days is also being used in the treatment of primary sclerosing cholangitis, post-ERCP bleeding, benign polyps, radio frequency ablation of intraductal lesions and rare complications like mirizzi syndrome (with cholangioscopic lithotripsy [35].

5. Percutaneous approaches

5.1 Percutaneous trans-hepatic cholangiography

PTC or Percutaneous trans-hepatic cholangiography is an invasive procedure commonly used for both diagnostic and therapeutic purposes. It involves the insertion of a needle into the biliary tract, followed by catheter placement for percutaneous transhepatic biliary drainage. Radio contrast is injected into one or more biliary ducts and possibly the duodenum, and is subsequently seen under fluoroscopic or ultrasound guidance. PTC is considered a pioneer in managing obstructive jaundice in malignancies, and it helps reduce bilirubin levels, improve liver function, and enable other treatments such as drainage and diagnostics.

5.2 Applications in complex biliary obstructions

Endoscopic Retrograde Cholangio-pancreatography (ERCP) is the mainstay treatment for managing biliary obstructions in patients with bilio-enteric anastomotic strictures (BEAS) and calculi. However, in patients who have undergone surgeries that distort the upper gastrointestinal (GI) anatomy (these include Billroth II distal gastrectomy, Roux-en-Y reconstruction bypass, pancreaticoduodenectomy, and hepaticojejunostomy), the biliary tree gets harder to access with an oral endoscopy, making ERCP more complicated. These procedures form BEAS that promote cholestasis, and their sutures are responsible for generating foreign body reactions that form calculi, thus worsening the biliary strictures. Furthermore, biliary sepsis and comorbidities make these patients poor candidates for surgical management, thus requiring the need for PTC [36].

Current guidance recommends percutaneous radiological stone extraction for patients for whom endoscopic procedures are contraindicated or unsuccessful. Biliary access is achieved by inserting a PTC drain *via* a catheter that performs necessary interventions under fluoroscopic guidance. This procedure is combined with lithotripsy, which uses the PTC biliary access for duct clearance under video cholangioscopy guidance, with lithotripsy that is needed for stone fragmentation [36].

PTC has also shown a better therapeutic success rate, less cholangitis and lower reintervention rate as compared to ERCP in cases of biliary drainage in malignant hilar biliary strictures.

PTC has also been reported to be useful in complex cases of foreign body impaction. Dormia basket is an instrument often used in the endoscopic removal of stones from the common bile duct, as seen in cases of choledocholithiasis. However, in cases when the stone size is massive, there is a higher probability of impaction of Dormia basket (DB) in the common bile duct. Due to the complexity of the case, a parallel approach requiring PTC and drainage with simultaneous endoscopy is required to safely remove the impacted foreign body. The sole use of ERCP in such cases resulted in severing of the holding wires, making the retrieval of the DB difficult. This can further be complicated by the perforation of CBD by the metallic tip of DB, thus requiring PTC to remove the DB as well as to enable drainage of the perforated CBD [37].

5.3 PTC with percutaneous transhepatic biliary drainage (PTBD) after kasai portoenterostomy

Kasai Portoenterostomy (KP) is a standard procedure done in patients diagnosed with biliary atresia. After the procedure, patients with biliary atresia(BA) occasionally develop complications, including recurrent cholangitis, biliary stricture, and cystic dilatation of the intrahepatic bile duct. This procedure has been tried in adult patients with BA with native livers, although the procedure has shown some success in reducing the frequency of complications, this procedure is not recommended to be performed easily on these patients because of a low success rate [38].

5.4 PTC with PTBD in hilar cholangiocarcinoma

Hilar Cholangiocarcinoma (hCCA) is a primary tumour of the biliary tract associated with a poor prognosis. Due to its anatomical origin and characteristics, it most commonly presents with painless obstructive jaundice. Depending on the staging, both therapeutic and palliative care measures can be taken. Compared to endoscopic drainage, the use of PTC with PTBD has the advantage that a specific duct can be targeted for treatment and to maximise the drainage from the remaining functional parenchyma. It has been shown to be more effective in reducing post-procedure complications like cholangitis and helps in better priming of the surgery.

The choice of procedure in a therapeutic setting mainly depends on the type of procedure performed. Patients with Bismuth II have been reported to perform better with ERCP, while patients who have undergone Bismuth IIIa or IV and have a bilirubin level greater than 8.8 mg/dl reported better results with initial PTBD [39].

When attending to patients requiring palliative care, one should keep in mind that the end goal of a procedure in such patients is to improve their quality of life. PTC with PTBD, which allows for the placement of an external stent, has shown a better quality of life after PTBD as compared to ERCP. A potential cause for this result is the higher incidence of post-procedural fever in groups undergoing endoscopic biliary stenting. Another benefit of this procedure is that percutaneous tenting can be done, eliminating the burden of caring for an external drainage tube for the rest of the patient's life [39].

5.5 Ablation techniques

The percutaneous modalities that are available today include the radiofrequency ablation(RFA), microwave ablation(MWA), cryoablation, irreversible electroporation, laser and high intensity focused ultrasound. In this chapter RFA and MWA will be primarily discussed.

Biliary tumours, namely cholangiocarcinoma, present with a high mortality rate and a poor prognosis. Traditionally treated by surgical resection, these tumours at the time of diagnosis are often not surgical candidates due to the high tumour burden and associated comorbidities. In addition to this, there is a very high tumour recurrence rate after resection. In such cases, percutaneous ablation techniques as mentioned above have proven to be beneficial.

5.6 RFA

Radiofrequency ablation works by generating an area of necrosis within the targeted tissue by applying thermal therapy *via* an electrode that provides an alternating current, causing ions to reverberate rapidly, thus increasing tissue temperature. The thermal energy produced induces a coagulative necrosis and subsequent death of malignant cells. This helps in completely eradicating the tumour at the same time preserving the remaining healthy tissue. RFA has also been shown to improve the survival and the quality of life in patients with unresectable cholangiocarcinoma. It does so by maintaining biliary drainage by tumour ablation within the biliary ducts or occluded metallic stents [40].

RFA can be approached in numerous ways, including surgical, percutaneous, and, more recently, the endoscopic modality. There have been advances in this technique to prevent excessive heating and collateral damage to the surrounding tissues. This was achieved by developing a specialised catheter named endo luminal radiofrequency ablation fitted with an automatic temperature probe to detect overheating. The advancement in ERCP has allowed the concomitant use of RFA to achieve stepwise ablation of the diseased tissues. RFA, however, has it is fair share of limitations; the therapeutic efficacy of this procedure is inversely related to the tumour size and its location. It is difficult to carry out this procedure in tumours in close approximation

Radio frequency ablation	Microwave ablation
1. Causes coagulative tissue necrosis using thermal energy from an electrode providing alternate current	1. Works by depositing energy into tissues using frictional heat generated from electromagnetic radiation induced rotation of mainly water molecules.
2. Lower ablative temperatures reached near blood vessels due to "heat sink" effects	2. Higher ablative temperatures reached due to low susceptibility of heat sink effect
3. Slower as compared to MWA in time taken to reach optimum temperature	3. Faster as compared to RFA to reach optimum ablative temperatures
4. Lesser efficacy in charred desiccated tissue and also lesser efficiency in lung and bones	4. Better than RFA in charred tissue, lung and bones

Table 3.
Evaluating the differences: Radiofrequency ablation vs. microwave ablation [40, 41].

to large vessels as the cooling effect of flowing blood can result in a "heat sink" effect, which results in the inability to reach maximal temperatures and henceforth causes incomplete cell destruction. RFA is also contraindicated in patients who are pregnant and those having cardiac devices or disorders of coagulopathy [40].

5.7 MWA

Microwave ablation is another percutaneous ablation technique commonly used in biliary tract diseases and has emerged as a suitable alternative for RFA. This technique has been shown to overcome many limitations of RFA. MWA works by depositing energy into tissues through electromagnetic radiation-induced rotation of dipole molecules, like water, which results in the formation of frictional heat. MWA generates higher temperatures as compared to RFA in a shorter time, leading to larger ablation zones and comparatively lesser susceptibility to heat sink effects of adjacent blood vessels. MWA is also proven to be more effective in tissues that have high impedance, such as charred desiccated tissue (**Table 3**) [41].

5.8 Outcomes of ablative techniques in cholangiocarcinoma

The treatment of cholangiocarcinoma depends on its anatomical location and resectability. At present, RFA is mainly employed for extrahepatic cholangiocarcinoma, it is use in cases of intrahepatic cholangiocarcinoma has limitations, but can be achieved by using ERCP or endoscopic ultrasound (EUS). Multiple studies have shown the efficacy of RFA in the treatment of cholangiocarcinoma and stent patency [40].

MWA in the current times has shown to take over RFA in treatment procedures, similarly to RFA, MWA has shown to be efficacious in reducing mortality rate and has proven to show better prognosis in patients with cholangiocarcinoma [41].

6. Minimally invasive techniques

6.1 Laparoscopic advancements

The recent advances in minimally invasive surgery have changed the entire face of abdominal surgery. Since the 1990's laparoscopic surgery has been the treatment of choice for cholecystectomy. These procedures have witnessed major advances with the coming of robotic surgery. These procedures have the advantages of minimal wound extension, early post-operative recovery, and fewer post-operative complications. To cover these advancements, newly enhanced imaging techniques such as high-definition cameras and fluorescence imaging with newer laparoscopic instruments and techniques will be discussed under this section.

6.2 Enhanced imaging technologies

The major limitation of laparoscopic surgery is the inability to perceive adequate depth. Since the foundation of laparoscopic surgery, there have been various advances focussing on increasing the quality of image and depth perception. The current preferred endovision technology is the regular high-definition (HD) system having a resolution of 1080 pixels. To overcome the mentioned problem, a 3D endovision system was designed. The latest generation high-definition 3D technology has also effectively minimised the surgeon's post-procedural related headaches, dizziness, and vomiting. The use of 3D technology is associated with both shortened operative time and a significant reduction in complication rate. Recently, there has also been a development of ultra-high-definition to improve the depth perception in surgery. The 4 K technology, which is primarily an extension of the existing two-dimensional working environment, uses a robust resolution of 3840 x 2160 pixels. The higher quality of imaging provides the operating surgeon with a larger image of the operative field. It provides a monocular depth perception by virtue of indirect visual cues, shadows of the structures, motion parallax, colour, and contrast of the operative field. This technology has also been found useful in reducing the intra-operative blood loss as well as the operating time. Other advantages of this system include a 5 mm angled optic that is easy to rotate for a wider view of the operating field and no requirement to wear polarised glasses during surgery, thus making it an efficient alternative to 3D technology [42].

Fluorescence imaging-Near-Infrared (NIR) fluorescence imaging technique is a widely adopted real-time imaging used in surgery in various clinical fields. To find the most appropriate fluorophore, many clinical studies were conducted, and this led to the discovery of Indocyanine green (ICG), which is now well known to be a harmless and appropriate fluorophore. ICG emits a fluorescence that peaks at a wavelength of approximately 840 nm, illuminated by the NIR light. It is barely influenced by water or haemoglobin and has been widely used as a suitable fluorophore in biliary systems. With advancements in the fields of minimally invasive procedures, attaining ICG imaging has become relatively more simplified, however, there are still several barriers, including the high cost of the essential camera system and high discrepancies between real and fusion images that have to be overcome. Recent investigations to verify the effectiveness of another fluorophore, namely sodium fluorescein (SF) have been conducted in porcine models. Under exposure to blue light, SF has the ability to emit a green light at the wavelengths of 520–530 nm to penetrate thin tissue. In contrast with the NIR fluorescence technique using ICG, this blue light fluorescence does not require an expensive camera system, as the light can be visualised by the conventional laparoscopic system. Furthermore, it provides the benefit to visualise the tracer and surrounding tissues without having any discrepancies regarding real-time and fusion images, thus paving the way for a more optimal fluorophore in SF as compared to ICG [43].

6.3 New laparoscopic techniques

With the rapid development of minimally invasive techniques through meticulous approaches, new laparoscopic methods are continuously being introduced. Although laparoscopic procedure poses challenges like restrictions of movement in the operating field and use of pedals for controlling the operating system, many new surgical methods, instruments, and devices have been developed to improve the working conditions that would help enhance the dexterity and accuracy during the required procedure. The newer methods include, Natural Orifice Transluminal Endoscopic Surgery (NOTES), Single Incision Laparoscopic Procedure (SILS), Robot-Assisted Laparoscopic Surgery (RALS), and Fluorescence-Guided Laparoscopic Surgery [44].

Natural orifice transluminal endoscopic surgery (NOTES). As the name suggests, this technique utilises access to the peritoneal cavity through natural orifices without any incisions or without passing through the anterior abdominal wall. This procedure is performed with existing endoscopic techniques using instruments in one body cavity, usually the peritoneal cavity. This access can be attained by passing an endoscope through a natural orifice such as the mouth, anus, vagina, or urethra and/or sometimes through incisions to create internal orifices. A combination of NOTES with a direct transcutaneous entry to the peritoneal cavity using the laparoscopic equipment is called HYBRID NOTES. Since these techniques eliminate the need for external incisions, it has potential benefits such as reduced post-operative pain, faster recovery time, and improved cosmesis. Although NOTES is still in its experimental stage, it holds great promise in procedures like cholecystectomy [44].

Single incision laparoscopic procedure (SILS): This procedure involves the use of laparoscopic techniques through a single small incision that is usually present at the umbilicus. As the port counts are consolidated into one single incision, it has proven to show many advantages over the traditional laparoscopic procedure. Benefits include decreased discomfort and pain, faster recovery period, superior cosmetic outcomes, and fewer port-associated complications [44].

Fluorescence-guided laparoscopic surgery: As mentioned earlier, it uses a fluorophore, mainly ICG, to enhance the visualisation of anatomical structures and pathological tissues during surgery. Fluorescence imaging allows surgeons to accurately identify and delineate critical structures, such as blood vessels and tumours, reducing the risk of intra-operative complications.

6.4 Robot-assisted laparoscopic surgery (RALS)

A surgical robot is primarily a computer-controlled system used to assist the surgeon during a procedure. Originally planned to be used in the process of telesurgery, it has shown great prowess in the operating theatre to facilitate laparoscopic surgery.

6.4.1 Benefits of RALS

- Improved orientation and dexterity, especially when a procedure requires suturing in small spaces or facilitating ergonomic instruments at angles.
- There is an availability of numerous instrumental tips for the laparoscopic instrument.
- Helps in better three-dimensional visualisation as well as tremor reduction.
- Improved survival, lesser blood loss, less post-operative pain, better cosmesis, and a faster return to physical activity as compared to open surgery.
- Compared to the traditional laparoscopic procedure, RALS has a shorter learning curve, and thus, surgeons can be trained faster in this technique [44, 45].

6.4.2 Challenges of RALS

- Reduced flexibility
- Requires increased operative time
- This procedure is more expensive as compared to the other laparoscopic procedures.

- RALS cholecystectomy has been shown to be associated with a higher risk of bile duct injury necessitating a definitive operative repair within 1 year. There is also a higher chance of biliary interventions and serious complications [44–46].

7. Gene therapy and regenerative medicine

7.1 Gene therapy

Advancements in research have demonstrated that gene therapy is being used more often to treat biliary tract disorders. Pathological processes such as fibrosis are involved in diseases like Primary biliary cholangitis (PBC) and Primary sclerosing cholangitis (PSC), which can lead to end-stage liver failure. Liver transplants are often used in conjunction with the above-mentioned illnesses to treat additional cholangiopathies that have lethal consequences. However, developments in gene therapy facilitate the management of these ailments. Rodent models are still being used to study these treatments.

The renin-angiotensin system, which is important for blood pressure management and sodium-water balance as well as tissue healing, is the target of the therapies. According to scientific data, angiotensin II (Ang II) is the causative agent of hepatic and biliary fibrosis. An intraperitoneal injection of an adeno-associated viral vector (AAV) containing the gene encoding for angiotensin-converting enzyme 2 (ACE2) was used. The viral genome is integrated into the cell by the process of transduction, which causes ACE2 expression to rise and Ang II levels to fall. This aids in limiting the amount of fibrosis that develops in the damaged tissue. Systemic adverse effects are a common occurrence with this therapy since it alters blood pressure and fluid and electrolyte balance [47].

The development of novel gene editing techniques like clustered regularly interspaced short palindromic repeats (CRISPR) allows for the study of genetic illnesses such as biliary atresia and Alagille syndrome.

7.2 Regenerative medicine

7.2.1 Cell therapy

In cell therapy, healthy tissue is used to harvest pluripotent or multipotent cells, which are then cultivated *in vitro* to produce the desired progeny. Liver transplantation is becoming less common as a substitute for cell therapy. Repopulating injured biliary system locations with stem/progenitor cells is the method used in these therapies [48]. Within the adult hepatic and biliary niches, there are two distinct

HpSCs	BTSCs
• Bipotent progenitor cells	• Multipotent stem cells
• Located within the Canals of Hering.	• Located within the Peribiliary glands of Intrahepatic and extrahepatic bile ducts.
• Can differentiate into mature hepatocytes and cholangiocytes	• Can differentiate into hepatic and pancreatic lineages

Table 4.
Differences between hepatic stem/progenitor cells (HpSCs) and biliary tree stem/progenitor cells (BTSCs) [49].

populations of stem/progenitor cells: hepatic stem/progenitor cells (HpSCs) and biliary tree stem/progenitor cells (BTSCs) (**Table 4**).

Acute hepatitis, viral cirrhosis, alcoholic steatohepatitis, non-alcoholic fatty liver disease, and cholangiopathies are among the illnesses associated with the HpSCs lineage. Primary sclerosing cholangitis, cholangiocarcinoma, non-anastomotic strictures, and biliary atresia are among the illnesses associated with the BTSCs lineage. The two stem cell lineages are rarely employed in the homeostatic regeneration necessary for the physiological make-or-break of the tissue, despite the fact that they can both activate in response to harm. This is because mature hepatocytes have a large capacity for regeneration. The hepatic and biliary tract's disease circumstances stimulate stem cells through many signalling pathways.

On the other hand, biliary tract diseases cause cell injury that is the primary cause of BTSC activation, despite their presence in close proximity to the biliary tree. BTSCs proliferate and remodel extensively in lesions of primary sclerosing cholangitis, resulting in the formation of dysplastic or hyperplastic glands surrounding the biliary systems. They also release angiogenic and proinflammatory factors, which aid in the process of fibrogenesis, or scarring. Additionally, pre-neoplastic lesions that eventually turn into cholangiocarcinoma are formed by BTSCs [49]. Research is still being done to gather stronger proof of the value of cell treatment in biliary diseases that affect the extrahepatic and intrahepatic liver [48].

7.2.2 Tissue engineering

Organoids are *in vitro*-cultivated, basic organ tissues made from stem cells. Organoids are generated from biliary epithelial cells, also known as cholangiocytes, specifically for the bile ducts. The functional abilities of cholangiocytes are restricted based on the site of extraction. Cholangiocytes lose their unique capabilities as they become organoids, however, these can be recovered *in vitro* by giving the organoids environmental cues. While organoids can regenerate damaged tissue and restore organ function, this ability is limited to *in vitro* experiments. *In vivo* outcomes from animal research have been somewhat lacking [50].

8. Conclusion

The traditional methods of treating biliary diseases have room for improvement. While adjuvant therapy has shown significant potential in improving patient outcomes. These advances hold promise not only for improving patient outcomes but also for reducing the need for invasive diagnostic procedures, ultimately leading to a less burdensome healthcare experience for patients. Certain approaches, such as targeted therapies, show promise by directly attacking the underlying causes of cancer, which may increase the chances of eradication. This has been made possible by ongoing research in gene therapy is paving the way for a deeper understanding of the genetic factors involved in biliary diseases, which could lead to the development of more personalised treatments. The use of prophylactic antibiotics and ensuring effective pain management can accelerate recovery and enhance the overall quality of care by lowering the risk of post-operative systemic complications. Additionally, employing minimally invasive techniques can further improve the quality of care. Furthermore, advancements in regenerative medicine offer the potential to reduce the need for liver transplantation by promoting the regeneration of damaged liver tissue.

A combined effort by the physicians, surgeons, and other stakeholders to venture into further research on these new modalities and integrate them with the traditional methods could improve patient outcomes and quality of life.

Acknowledgements

The author acknowledges the use of OpenAI's ChatGPT and grammerly for language polishing, reviewing and confirming the headings.

Author details

Sree Harshitha Vallabhaneni*, Sri Sravya Lalitha Chandrika Thungathurthi, Prem Kurra and Supraj Teeparthy
Apollo Institute of Medical Sciences and Research, Hyderabad, India

*Address all correspondence to: harshithabangaaru@gmail.com

References

[1] Hodler J, Kubik-Huch RA, von Schulthess GK, editors. Diseases of the Abdomen and Pelvis 2018-2021: Diagnostic Imaging - IDKD Book. Cham, CH: Springer; 2018

[2] Lowenfels AB, Maisonneuve P. Pancreatico-biliary malignancy: Prevalence and risk factors. Annals of Oncology. 1999;**10**:S1-S3. DOI: 10.1093/annonc/10.suppl_4.s1 [Accessed: 17 May 2022]

[3] Khan ZR et al. Risk factors for biliary tract cancers. American Journal of Gastroenterology. 1999;**94**(1):149-152. DOI: 10.1111/j.1572-0241.1999.00786.x [Accessed: 1 November 2022]

[4] Jiang Y, Jiang L, Li F, et al. The epidemiological trends of biliary tract cancers in the United States of America. BMC Gastroenterology. 2022;**22**:546. DOI: 10.1186/s12876-022-02637-8

[5] Torre LA et al. Worldwide burden of and trends in mortality from gallbladder and other biliary tract cancers. Clinical Gastroenterology and Hepatology. 2018;**16**(3):427-437. DOI: 10.1016/j.cgh.2017.08.017 [Accessed: 26 February 2020]

[6] Hennedige TP et al. Imaging of malignancies of the biliary tract- an update. Cancer Imaging: The Official Publication of the International Cancer Imaging Society. 2014;**14**(1):14. Available from: www.ncbi.nlm.nih.gov/pmc/articles/PMC4331820/. DOI: 10.1186/1470-7330-14-14

[7] Swensson J, Zaheer A, Conwell D, Sandrasegaran K, Manfredi R, Tirkes T. Secretin-enhanced MRCP: How and why-*AJR* expert panel narrative review. AJR. American Journal of Roentgenology. 2021;**216**(5):1139-1149. DOI: 10.2214/AJR.20.24857

[8] Mazroua JA, Almalki YE, Alaa M, et al. Precision mapping of intrahepatic biliary anatomy and its anatomical variants having a normal liver using 2D and 3D MRCP. Diagnostics (Basel). 2023;**13**(4):726. Published 2023 Feb 14. DOI: 10.3390/diagnostics13040726

[9] Cui XY, Chen HW. Role of diffusion-weighted magnetic resonance imaging in the diagnosis of extrahepatic cholangiocarcinoma. World Journal of Gastroenterology. 2010;**16**(25):3196-3201. DOI: 10.3748/wjg.v16.i25.3196

[10] Xu HX. Contrast-enhanced ultrasound in the biliary system: Potential uses and indications. World Journal of Radiology. 2009;**1**(1):37-44. DOI: 10.4329/wjr.v1.i1.37), 10.4329/wjr.v1.i1.37

[11] Lee NK, Kim S, Kim GH, et al. Diffusion-weighted imaging of biliopancreatic disorders: Correlation with conventional magnetic resonance imaging. World Journal of Gastroenterology. 2012;**18**(31):4102-4117. DOI: 10.3748/wjg.v18.i31.4102

[12] Lu RC, She B, Gao WT, et al. Positron-emission tomography for hepatocellular carcinoma: Current status and future prospects. World Journal of Gastroenterology. 2019;**25**(32):4682-4695. DOI: 10.3748/wjg.v25.i32.4682

[13] Wagner ES, Abdelgawad HAH, Landry M, Asfour B, Slidell MB, Azzam R. Use of shear wave elastography for the diagnosis and follow-up of biliary atresia: A meta-analysis. World Journal of Gastroenterology. 2022;**28**(32):4726-4740. DOI: 10.3748/wjg.v28.i32.4726

[14] Nakaura T, Kobayashi N, Yoshida N, et al. Update on the use of artificial

intelligence in hepatobiliary MR imaging. Magnetic Resonance in Medical Sciences. 2023;**22**(2):147-156. DOI: 10.2463/mrms.rev.2022-0102. In cases where subtle abnormalities might be overlooked, AI can flag areas of concern for further review, particularly in complex biliary anatomy

[15] Mervak BM, Fried JG, Wasnik AP. A review of the clinical applications of artificial intelligence in abdominal imaging. Diagnostics. 2023;**13**(18):2889. DOI: 10.3390/diagnostics13182889

[16] Li YC, Li KS, Liu ZL, et al. Research progress of bile biomarkers and their immunoregulatory role in biliary tract cancers. Frontiers in Immunology. 2022;**13**(28):1049812. DOI: 10.3389/fimmu.2022.1049812 [Accessed: 31 August 2024]

[17] Macias RIR, Banales JM, Sangro B, et al. The search for novel diagnostic and prognostic biomarkers in cholangiocarcinoma. Biochimica et Biophysica Acta (BBA) - Molecular Basis of Disease. 2018;**1864**(4, Part B):1468-1477. DOI: 10.1016/j.bbadis.2017.08.002

[18] Yıldırım HÇ, Kavgaci G, Chalabiyev E, Dizdar O. Advances in the early detection of hepatobiliary cancers. Cancers. 2023;**15**(15):3880. DOI: 10.3390/cancers15153880

[19] García P et al. Current and new biomarkers for early detection, prognostic stratification, and management of gallbladder cancer patients. Cancer. 2020;**12**(12):3670-3670. Available from: www.ncbi.nlm.nih.gov/pmc/articles/PMC7762341/. DOI: 10.3390/cancers12123670 [Accessed: 28 July 2023]

[20] Proskuriakova E, Khedr A. Current targeted therapy options in the treatment of cholangiocarcinoma: A literature review. Cureus. 2022;**14**(6):e26233. Published 2022 Jun 23. DOI: 10.7759/cureus.26233

[21] Westphal JF, Brogard JM. Biliary tract infections: A guide to drug treatment. Drugs. 1999;**57**(1):81-91. DOI: 10.2165/00003495-199957010-00007

[22] Sharara AI, El Hajj II, Mroueh M, et al. Prophylaxis with ertapenem in patients with obstructive jaundice undergoing endoscopic retrograde cholangiopancreatography: Safety, efficacy, and biliary penetration. Southern Medical Journal. 2011;**104**(3):189-194. DOI: 10.1097/SMJ.0b013e318205de10

[23] Lammert F, Gurusamy K, Ko CW, et al. Gallstones. Nature Reviews. Disease Primers. 2016;**2**:16024. Published 2016 Apr 28. DOI: 10.1038/nrdp.2016.24

[24] Shaffer EA. Epidemiology and risk factors for gallstone disease: Has the paradigm changed in the 21st century? Current Gastroenterology Reports. 2005;**7**(2):132-140. DOI: 10.1007/s11894-005-0051-8

[25] Jiang B, Ye S. Pharmacotherapeutic pain management in patients undergoing laparoscopic cholecystectomy: A review. Advances in Clinical and Experimental Medicine. 2022;**31**(11):1275-1288. DOI: 10.17219/acem/151995

[26] Sarcognato S, Sacchi D, Grillo F, et al. Autoimmune biliary diseases: Primary biliary cholangitis and primary sclerosing cholangitis. Pathologica. 2021;**113**(3):170-184. DOI: 10.32074/1591-951X-245

[27] European Association for the Study of the Liver. Electronic address: easloffice@easloffice.eu; European Association for the Study of the Liver.

EASL clinical practice guidelines: The diagnosis and management of patients with primary biliary cholangitis. Journal of Hepatology. 2017;**67**(1):145-172. DOI: 10.1016/j.jhep.2017.03.022

[28] Chung SW, Lee JH, Kim MA, et al. Additional fibrate treatment in UDCA-refractory PBC patients. Liver International. 2019;**39**(9):1776-1785. DOI: 10.1111/liv.14165

[29] Floreani A, De Martin S. Treatment of primary sclerosing cholangitis. Digestive and Liver Disease. 2021;**53**(12):1531-1538. DOI: 10.1016/j.dld.2021.04.028

[30] Almuhaidb A, Olson D, Aadam AA. Advancements in endoscopic biliary interventions by gastroenterology. Semin Intervent Radiol. 2021;**38**(3):280-290. DOI: 10.1055/s-0041-1731266

[31] Daurka J, Loh A, Bird R, Howard A. A new laparoscopic technique: Suction removal of spilled gallstones. Annals of the Royal College of Surgeons of England. 2006;**88**(7):678-679. DOI: 10.1308/rcsann.2006.88.7.678b

[32] Vergunst H, Terpstra OT, Brakel K, Laméris JS, van Blankenstein M, Schröder FH. Extracorporeal shockwave lithotripsy of gallstones. Possibilities and limitations. Annals of Surgery. 1989;**210**(5):565-575. DOI: 10.1097/00000658-198911000-00001

[33] Yang K, Sun W, Cui L, Zou Y, Wen C, Zeng R. Advances in functional coatings on biliary stents. Regenerative Biomaterials. 2024;**11**:rbae001. Published 2024 Jan 18. DOI: 10.1093/rb/rbae001

[34] Szary NM, Al-Kawas FH. Complications of endoscopic retrograde cholangiopancreatography: How to avoid and manage them. Gastroenterology and Hepatolpogy (N Y). 2013;**9**(8):496-504

[35] Mauro A, Mazza S, Scalvini D, Lusetti F, Bardone M, Quaretti P, et al. The role of cholangioscopy in biliary diseases. Diagnostics. 2023;**13**(18):2933. DOI: 10.3390/diagnostics13182933

[36] Alabraba E, Travis S, Beckingham I. Percutaneous transhepatic cholangioscopy and lithotripsy in treating difficult biliary ductal stones: Two case reports. World Journal of Gastroenterology Endoscopy. 2019;**11**(4):298-307. DOI: 10.4253/wjge.v11.i4.298

[37] Misbahuddin-Leis M, Ankolvi M, Mishra M, et al. Unlocking the enigma: Combined percutaneous-transhepatic and endoscopic strategies for retrieval of severed Dormia basket in choledocholithiasis. A case report and literature review. Radiology Case Reports. 2024;**19**(7):2745-2750. Published 2024 Apr 19. DOI: 10.1016/j.radcr.2024.03.074

[38] Onishi Y, Shimizu H, Ohno T, et al. Percutaneous transhepatic biliary intervention in adult biliary atresia patients after kasai portoenterostomy. JPGN Reports. 2022;**3**(2):e206. Published 2022 May 9. DOI: 10.1097/PG9.0000000000000206

[39] Mocan T, Horhat A, Mois E, et al. Endoscopic or percutaneous biliary drainage in hilar cholangiocarcinoma: When and how? World Journal of Gastrointestinal Oncology. 2021;**13**(12):2050-2063. DOI: 10.4251/wjgo.v13.i12.2050

[40] Hendriquez R, Keihanian T, Goyal J, Abraham RR, Mishra R, Girotra M. Radiofrequency ablation in the management of primary hepatic and biliary tumors. World

Journal of Gastrointestinal Oncology. 2022;**14**(1):203-215. DOI: 10.4251/wjgo.v14.i1.203

[41] Sweeney J, Parikh N, El-Haddad G, Kis B. Ablation of intrahepatic cholangiocarcinoma. Semin Intervent Radiol. 2019;**36**(4):298-302. DOI: 10.1055/s-0039-1696649

[42] Singla V, Bhattacharjee HK, Gupta E, Singh D, Mishra AK, Kumar D. Performance of three-dimensional and ultra-high-definition (4K) technology in laparoscopic surgery: A systematic review and meta-analysis. Journal of Minimally Invasive Surgery. 2022;**18**(2):167-175. DOI: 10.4103/jmas.jmas_122_21

[43] Kim S, Lee CM, Lee Y, Han HJ, Song TJ. Laparoscopic fluorescence imaging technique for visualizing biliary structures using sodium fluorescein: The result of a preclinical study in a porcine model. Annals of Surgical Treatment and Research. 2023;**104**(3):144-149. DOI: 10.4174/astr.2023.104.3.144

[44] Basunbul LI, Alhazmi LSS, Almughamisi SA, Aljuaid NM, Rizk H, Moshref R. Recent technical developments in the field of laparoscopic surgery: A literature review. Cureus. 2022;**14**(2):e22246. Published 2022 Feb 15. DOI: 10.7759/cureus.22246

[45] Lee WJ, Chan CP, Wang BY. Recent advances in laparoscopic surgery. Asian Journal of Endoscopic Surgery. 2013;**6**(1):1-8. DOI: 10.1111/ases.12001

[46] Kalata S, Thumma JR, Norton EC, Dimick JB, Sheetz KH. Comparative safety of robotic-assisted vs laparoscopic cholecystectomy. JAMA Surgery. 2023;**158**(12):1303-1310. DOI: 10.1001/jamasurg.20

[47] Rajapaksha IG, Angus PW, Herath CB. Current therapies and novel approaches for biliary diseases. World Journal of Gastrointestinal Pathophysiology. 2019;**10**(1):1-10. DOI: 10.4291/wjgp.v10.i1.1

[48] Kurial SNT, Willenbring H. Emerging cell therapy for biliary diseases. Science. 2021;**371**(6531):786-787. DOI: 10.1126/science.abg3179

[49] Overi D, Carpino G, Cardinale V, Franchitto A, Safarikia S, Onori P, et al. Contribution of resident stem cells to liver and biliary tree regeneration in human diseases. International Journal of Molecular Sciences. 2018;**19**(10):2917. DOI: 10.3390/ijms19102917

[50] Sampaziotis F, Muraro D, Tysoe OC, et al. Cholangiocyte organoids can repair bile ducts after in the human liver. Science. 2021;**371**(6531):839-846. DOI: 10.1126/science.aaz6964

Chapter 6

Laparoscopic Cholecystectomy from the Classic Approach to Recent Updates

Mohie El-Din Mostafa Madany

Abstract

The current chapter provides a comprehensive overview of complications, difficult situations, and technical challenges related to laparoscopic cholecystectomy (LC). It revisited the classic approach, reviewing all the steps with the new advancements, and emphasizing the importance of preoperative imaging and intraoperative techniques for reducing complications. The chapter also discusses complex scenarios, including Mirizzi syndrome, cystic duct stones, GB mucocele, and acute cholecystitis, underlining tailored surgical approaches and the role of advanced imaging. It explores critical issues such as perforated GB, short or absent cystic duct, the seatbelt effect of the cystic artery, and strategies for managing frozen Calot's triangle, intrahepatic GB, cirrhotic liver, and morbid obesity during LC. The necessity of conversion to open surgery and the role of cholecystostomy, subtotal, completion, and repeat cholecystectomy in complex cases are examined. The chapter underscores optimizing patient outcomes through meticulous surgical planning and advanced techniques.

Keywords: laparoscopic cholecystectomy, complications, difficult situation, cholecysto-choledocho-lithiasis, advanced imaging, surgical planning

1. Introduction

Laparoscopic cholecystectomy (LC) is a minimally invasive surgical procedure for gallbladder (GB) removal that is widely recognized as the gold standard for GB disease treatment. The laparoscope, equipped with a camera, allows the surgeon to view the abdominal cavity on a monitor, ensuring precise and effective GB removal. The procedure offers several advantages over traditional open cholecystectomy, including reduced postoperative pain, shorter hospital stays, faster recovery times, and smaller scars. LC has revolutionized GB surgery since its introduction in the late 1980s, becoming the preferred method for managing conditions such as gallstones, GB inflammation, and abnormal GB function. Notably, the procedure boasts high success rates and lower complication risks, a testament to its safety and reliability in significantly improving patient outcomes and quality of life [1, 2].

2. Revisiting the classic approach for laparoscopic cholecystectomy

The classic approach for LC is the cornerstone for every subsequent modification.

2.1 Key principles

The four-port technique includes one umbilical, two lateral, and one epigastric port. The patient is in the supine position with the operating table in slight reverse Trendelenburg and left tilt, which aids in moving the intestines away from the surgical field and improving access to the GB [1, 2].

2.2 Port placement

A 10–12 mm umbilical port accommodates the laparoscope. A 10 mm epigastric port below the xiphoid hosts dissecting instruments, a clip applier, and scissors. Right midclavicular and right anterior axillary ports, both 5 mm, assist in dissection and retraction [1, 2].

2.3 Procedure

Carbon dioxide insufflation (12–15 mmHg) establishes pneumoperitoneum, enhancing visibility. Achieving *the critical view of safety (CVS)* prevents bile duct injuries. It involves identifying the cystic duct and artery, ensuring that only two structures enter the GB before clipping and cutting [3, 4]. Grasping the GB fundus and retracting it toward the right shoulder while laterally retracting the infundibulum exposes Calot's triangle, cystic duct, and artery. Careful dissection within Calot's triangle ensures unambiguous identification of the cystic structures. Following critical view confirmation, cystic duct and artery clipping (with subsequent division) occur, typically with two clips on the ductal side and one on the GB side. Electrocautery or ultrasonic energy devices detach the GB from the liver bed, minimizing bleeding and liver injury. Post-detachment, the GB is placed in an endoscopic retrieval bag and extracted through the epigastric or the umbilical port to minimize peritoneal cavity contamination. Hemostasis is ensured through irrigation, and any residual bile or blood is aspirated. Finally, pneumoperitoneum release precedes port removal, with the closure of the fascia by absorbable sutures and the skin with nonabsorbable sutures as proline [1, 2].

2.4 Critique

Laparoscopic cholecystectomy has significant advantages over open cholecystectomy, including reduced postoperative pain, shorter recovery times, and minimal scarring. However, despite that and its widespread acceptance and success, several critiques and limitations are associated with the classic laparoscopic approach. First, in classic LC, the risk of bile duct injury, albeit rare (0.4–1.5%), looms large, potentially leading to bile leakage, infection, and additional surgeries. To mitigate this risk, techniques like intraoperative cholangiography and near-infrared fluorescence cholangiography are employed. However, technical challenges persist, demanding high surgical skill and experience due to limited visibility and range of motion, which may prolong operative times and increase complication risks. Postoperative discomfort, including incision site pain and referred shoulder pain from abdominal gas insufflation, adds to patient concerns. Efforts to alleviate these discomforts through methods like single-incision laparoscopic surgery (SILS) and robotic-assisted techniques show promise but await universal adoption [5–7].

2.5 Is the classic approach enough?

While the classic LC is highly effective and widely used, continuous advancements in surgical techniques and technologies hold promise for further improving patient outcomes [8]. In the next section, we will delve into the potential areas for improvement in LC, covering every step of the procedure.

3. Advancements in laparoscopic cholecystectomy

3.1 Perioperative preparation

Enhanced recovery after surgery (ERAS) protocols reduce hospital stays and improve recovery times. *Preoperatively*, ERAS emphasizes thorough patient education, updated fasting guidelines allowing clear fluids up to two hours before surgery, and carbohydrate loading to maintain energy levels and reduce insulin resistance. *Intraoperatively*, ERAS focuses on optimizing anesthesia and analgesia with multimodal strategies to minimize opioid use. *Postoperatively*, ERAS advocates for early mobilization and oral intake initiation to prevent complications such as deep vein thrombosis. Patients should drink clear fluids and eat light meals soon after surgery to stimulate gastrointestinal function and reduce ileus risk. Multimodal pain management continues to ensure effective relief. ERAS also includes prophylactic antibiotics, thromboprophylaxis, and strategies to reduce surgical site infections, with nutritional support tailored to promote healing [9, 10].

Improved imaging techniques, such as Magnetic Resonance Cholangiopancreatography (MRCP) and Endoscopic Ultrasound (EUS), can *stratify preoperative risk* by accurately identifying bile duct stones and anatomical variations, thus reducing intraoperative complications and improving outcomes [11, 12].

3.2 Anesthesia and patient positioning

Anesthesia innovations using total intravenous anesthesia (TIVA) and regional blocks improve postoperative pain management and patient recovery [13, 14]. *Trendelenburg positioning* is used to move the small intestine away from the pelvis, and *reverse Trendelenburg* is used to move the bowel away from the upper abdominal region. These adjustments enhance visibility and access to the GB, facilitating safer and more efficient surgical procedures by providing better exposure to the surgical field to improve visibility and access to the GB during surgery [15].

3.3 Initial access and pneumoperitoneum

The initial access by *the optical trocar* with direct visualization minimizes the risk of injury to intra-abdominal organs, a common concern during the blind insertion of traditional trocars. This approach benefits patients with previous abdominal surgeries or other conditions that may alter normal anatomy [16]. Recent studies suggest that using *a low-pressure pneumoperitoneum*, between 10 and 12 mmHg, can significantly benefit patients. This reduction is associated with less postoperative pain. It improves cardiovascular and respiratory outcomes [17].

3.4 Ports: Number, size, and place

A recent literature review stated that the standard LC has been modified by utilizing over 50 different technological variants [18].

Four-port modified techniques: One approach involves reducing port sizes from 10 to 5 mm or 5 to 3 or 2 mm to minimize the trocar site hernia while maintaining the same number of ports. Surgeons using a 5-mm telescope may reduce the umbilical port size, while those using a 5-mm clip applicator may downsize the epigastric trocar. Some even opt for 3-mm trocars. For ease of GB removal, surgeons often select a 10-mm trocar at the umbilical or epigastric site, as the GB is extracted through this trocar in an Endobag. Additionally, to enhance cosmetic results, some surgeons place all trocars below the bikini line without altering their size [18–20].

Three-port modified techniques: The most common method involves omitting the anterior axillary line port and using cranial traction on the GB fundus using a suture. Surgeons typically employ two 10-mm trocars and one 5-mm trocar, although some may use varying trocar sizes or even perform micro laparoscopic cholecystectomies with 3-mm trocars. An intriguing technique involves placing a traction suture on the GB, pulling the fundus toward the lower right chest area, and performing the cholecystectomy with just three ports. To prevent minor bile leakage during surgery, a figure-eight suture can be placed in the fundus, applying gentle traction to avoid rupturing the GB wall [21, 22].

The two-port modified technique demonstrates its versatility in various ways. Surgeons utilize two traction sutures with two ports, one in the fundus and the other in Hartmann's region of the GB. This technique can involve inserting traction sutures through the port or using specialized laparoscopic tools for traction. Notably, the instrument used for traction in the Hartmann's pouch can be inserted through the camera port. In some instances, the procedure is streamlined to just two incisions, with the umbilical port modified to a single port or a glove port, allowing the use of multiple instruments [18, 23].

Surgeons use the single-incision modified technique to access the abdomen from the belly button and insert all surgical equipment from the same location. Nonetheless, single-incision robot-assisted cholecystectomy examples have made their way into the literature. There are additional variations on the single incisions, so much so that gasless cases have been documented without CO2 injection [24].

In natural orifice transluminal endoscopic surgery (NOTES), hybrid transvaginal procedures are widely utilized, with the first trocar from the umbilical area and the remaining trocars transvaginal from the posterior fornix. One systematic review compared transvaginal NOTES with traditional laparoscopic surgery. Results showed no significant difference in intraoperative or postoperative complications between the two techniques. However, transvaginal NOTES patients experienced significantly less pain and had a shorter recovery time. Importantly, transvaginal NOTES is a safe and minimally invasive procedure, making it a recommended choice for cholecystectomy, adnexectomy, and appendectomy [25].

In needlescopic cholecystectomy, the surgeon utilizes very small-diameter instruments (2–3 mm) in contrast to the standard 5–10 mm instruments in smaller ports, leading to a significant reduction in the procedure's invasiveness. The primary advantages include cosmetic benefits due to less visible scarring, reduced postoperative pain, and a quicker recovery, all of which contribute to improved patient outcomes. Additionally, the smaller incisions lower the risk of wound infections. However, this technique presents technical challenges, requiring more skill and precision [26].

Angled scope cholecystectomy employing a 30-degree or 45-degree laparoscope provides a broader and more flexible field of view than the traditional straight laparoscope, which allows surgeons to see around corners and access structures not directly in line with the port. That is particularly beneficial for visualizing areas behind the GB or in the upper abdomen, facilitating precise dissection and tissue manipulation. However, it requires additional training and practice, as the altered perspective can be disorienting. The cost of angled scopes may be higher than the standard scopes. Despite these challenges, enhanced visualization and access can significantly improve outcomes [20].

3.5 Dissection and exposure

Dissection and exposure are pivotal stages in LC, where precision and clarity are paramount to avoid complications, especially bile duct injuries. *Fluorescent cholangiography*, a practical method that uses indocyanine green (ICG) dye to highlight bile ducts under near-infrared fluorescence, has gained attention. This method allows surgeons to—clearly—delineate the bile ducts during dissection. The ICG dye is administered intravenously before the procedure, and it selectively binds to bile, which then fluoresces under near-infrared light, providing a real-time, clear map of the bile ducts. The enhanced visualization also helps in detecting any anatomical variations [27].

Another significant development is using advanced *energy devices* such as the harmonic scalpel and LigaSure. These devices have revolutionized the approach to tissue dissection and hemostasis. The harmonic scalpel uses ultrasonic vibrations to cut and coagulate tissue simultaneously, providing precise dissection with minimal thermal spread, which is crucial in delicate areas like the Calot's triangle. Similarly, LigaSure employs bipolar energy to seal blood vessels and tissue bundles effectively, offering superior hemostasis and reducing the risk of bleeding. Using these devices enhances the efficiency of the dissection process and significantly reduces operating times, offering an optimistic outlook for potential time-saving benefits [18, 28].

In resource-constrained settings, the practical and effective use of bipolar electrocautery is a viable option. One prospective study of 120 patients aimed to validate the safety and feasibility of using bipolar electrocautery in LC (**Figure 1**). The findings revealed that there was no intraoperative bleeding from the cystic artery or the right hepatic artery and no visceral injuries. The success rate was 100%, with no need for

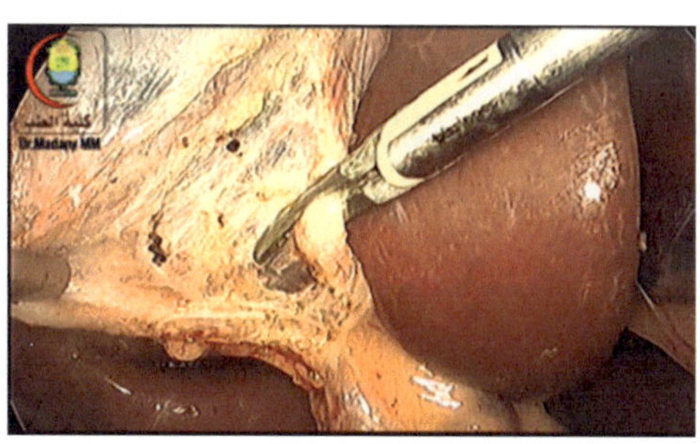

Figure 1.
The use of electrocautery in hemostatic control of the cystic artery in LC.

conversion. The results underscore that bipolar diathermy is a viable and effective method for hemostatic control of the cystic artery in LC [29].

3.6 Identifying and securing the cystic duct and artery

Emphasizing the achievement of *a Critical View of Safety (CVS)* has become standard to minimize the risk of bile duct injuries. Some surgeons also recommend routine intraoperative cholangiography for additional safety [30].

The Madany triangle technique (**Figure 2**), a novel and safe approach, places a high priority on achieving a Critical View of Safety (CVS) while significantly reducing the risk of extrahepatic biliary injury and bleeding. It strategically shifts the focus of dissection and cauterization away from the danger zones (the Calot triangle), specifically targeting the proximal part of the cystic duct at its junction with the GB neck. This approach effectively avoids the complications associated with any anatomical variation within the Calot triangle, as the Caterpillar hump of the right hepatic artery (**Figure 3**). The Madany et al. study provides robust evidence of the technique's effectiveness and safety. The early scarification of the cystic artery during GB skeletonization eliminates the seat belt effect of the artery and its branches on the proximal part of the GB, infundibulum, and cystic duct as shown in **Figure 3** and the attached video. The technique potentially reduces the incidence of bile duct injury and perioperative bleeding, ultimately improving patient outcomes [31].

In the clipless cholecystectomy, the metallic clips are replaced with alternative methods, such as ultrasonic dissection or suturing, to secure the cystic duct and artery. This transition aims to mitigate the risks associated with clip-related complications. Ultrasonic dissection provides precise and adequate hemostasis. This method

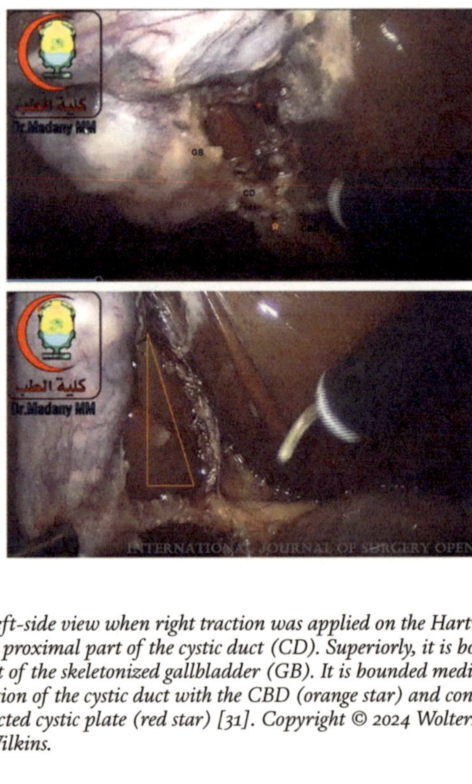

Figure 2.
Madani triangle from the left-side view when right traction was applied on the Hartman pouch; it is bounded laterally by the skeletonized proximal part of the cystic duct (CD). Superiorly, it is bounded by the posterior surface of the proximal part of the skeletonized gallbladder (GB). It is bounded medially by an imaginary line between a point at the junction of the cystic duct with the CBD (orange star) and continuous with a point at the anterior end of the dissected cystic plate (red star) [31]. Copyright © 2024 Wolters Kluwer. Published by Lippincott Williams and Wilkins.

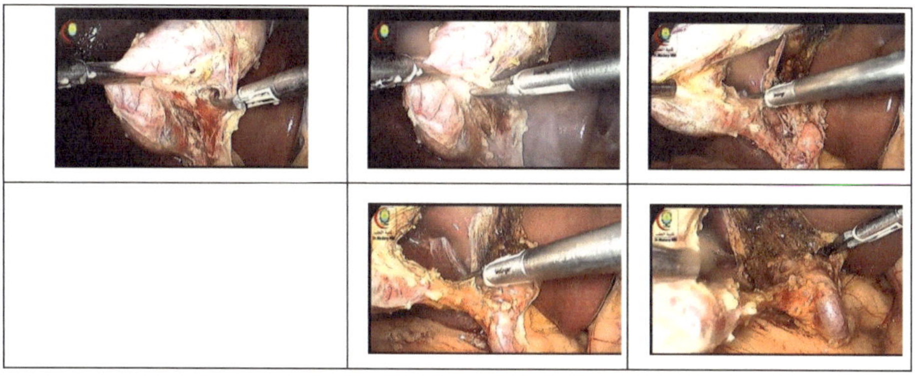

Figure 3.
Early scarification of the cystic artery during GB skeletonization eliminates the seat belt effect of the artery and its branches on the proximal part of the GB, infundibulum, and cystic duct.

reduces thermal spread to adjacent tissues and minimizes intraoperative bleeding. Additionally, suturing the cystic duct and artery offers a secure and reliable method of ligation, particularly in complex cases. The versatility of this method is particularly advantageous in patients with dense adhesions or distorted anatomy due to chronic inflammation or previous surgeries, providing a comprehensive solution. Advanced suturing techniques ensure a robust closure, significantly decreasing the likelihood of postoperative bile leaks. Moreover, eliminating foreign metallic objects from the surgical site enhances postoperative imaging and reduces the risk of long-term complications related to clip presence [32, 33].

In LC, securing the cystic duct can be achieved through various methods, such as *suturing ligation* (**Figure 4**), clips, electrocautery, and vessel sealing devices. Suturing ligation is highlighted as a safe and cost-effective option, especially in low-resource settings like developing countries. One study assessed the safety and feasibility of intracorporeal suturing ligation for cystic duct management. The mean time for cystic duct ligation was 3.03 minutes, and the procedure had a remarkable 100% success rate with no intraoperative bile duct injury, leakage, or bleeding. The technique demonstrated low rates of postoperative complications and did not require conversion. This underscores the method as a crucial skill in LC, essential for resource-constrained environments, and instills confidence in its effectiveness [34].

3.7 Gallbladder removal

Using an *endobag for GB retrieval* plays a critical role in maintaining a sterile surgical field during LC. Surgeons can effectively minimize the risk of bile spillage

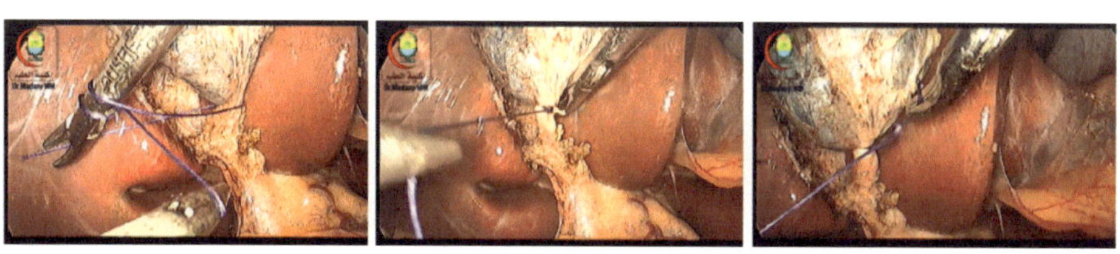

Figure 4.
Intracorporeal suturing ligation for cystic duct.

and subsequent complications, such as infection or peritoneal irritation, by securely containing the GB and any associated debris within the bag before extraction through the trocar site. This method ensures a clean and safe procedure. A systematic review, providing comprehensive insights, analyzed studies comparing endobag versus direct extraction techniques. The review's findings indicate that using an endobag significantly decreases the incidence of SSI and bile spillage compared to direct extraction. The incidence of intra-abdominal collection was comparable between both groups. However, the endobag method often necessitates a larger fascial defect for GB extraction, while no significant difference was observed in port site hernia rates [35].

A retrospective analysis aimed to evaluate the safety of GB retrieval through the right lumbar port using the 5-5-5-10 approach, with a focus on trocar site hernias (TSH) rates, has been published. The study meticulously reviewed records and operative videos of 977 patients who underwent LC at Aswan University Hospital's general surgery department. The results were striking; not a single instance of TSH was reported during the follow-up period, which averaged 28.5 ± 12 months. This finding, along with other favorable outcomes, particularly regarding cosmetic appearance, further supports the safety and efficacy of the endobag method [36].

3.8 Closing the incisions

Recent innovations in LC include the development of *advanced fascial closure devices* to enhance the closure of port site incisions with improved precision. They often incorporate features such as self-anchoring mechanisms or absorbable fixation. In a recent study, *Nasr fascial closure device* was evaluated for fascial closure in laparoscopic surgery. The median time for complete closure of the port site was 63.0 seconds (interquartile range 76.8 seconds). Notably, no cases of TSH were reported during the 12–15-month follow-up period. The findings conclude that the novel device provides a safe, rapid, and effective port site closure technique [37].

Novel suturing techniques in LC focus on optimizing the closure of port site incisions through innovative stitching patterns or materials. Techniques such as barbed sutures, knotless closures, or extracorporeal knots (as in Madany closure) have gained attention for their ability to simplify the suturing process and enhance wound closure strength. These advancements aim to minimize tissue trauma, reduce operative time, and promote faster healing with improved cosmetic outcomes. A prospective study evaluated the Madany closure technique (**Figure 5**) for port site closure. The method demonstrated a median closure time of 83.5 seconds (interquartile range 44.75 seconds), indicating rapid closure. Notably, no TSH occurred during the 6-month follow-up period, underscoring the technique's safety and effectiveness [38, 39].

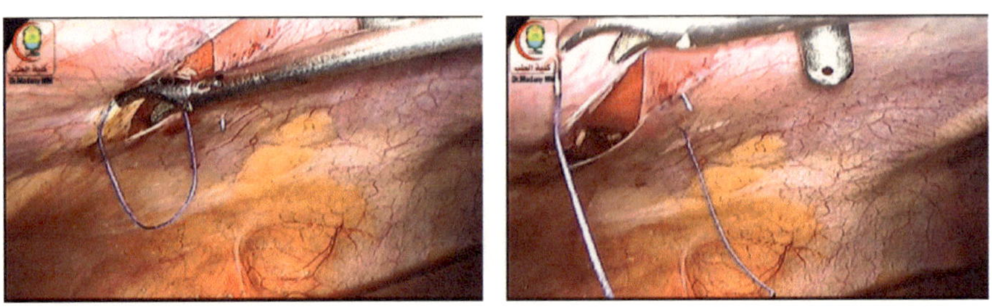

Figure 5.
Madany closure technique.

3.9 Postoperative care

Postoperative care in LC emphasizes *early mobilization and progressive diet advancement* as integral components of ERAS protocols. Early ambulation is typically initiated within hours of surgery. Likewise, the rapid advancement of diet from clear fluids to solid foods helps to diminish the postoperative ileus and allows for the recovery of normal gastrointestinal function sooner [9, 10].

Effective pain management in LC involves the implementation of multimodal analgesia strategies aimed at reducing opioid consumption while ensuring adequate pain relief. Multimodal analgesia combines various medications and techniques to target different pain pathways, thereby enhancing efficacy and minimizing side effects. Non-steroidal anti-inflammatory drugs (NSAIDs) and acetaminophen serve as cornerstone agents in this approach, providing adjunctive pain relief and reducing the need for opioids. Regional anesthesia techniques such as transversus abdominis plane (TAP) blocks or local anesthetic infiltration at trocar sites further contribute to localized pain control, enhancing patient comfort during the immediate postoperative period. This comprehensive pain management strategy supports the goals of ERAS protocols [40, 41].

3.10 Emerging technologies and techniques

Robotic surgical systems are at the forefront of revolutionizing minimally invasive surgery, particularly in single-port cholecystectomies. These systems offer a significant leap forward in surgical precision and safety with three-dimensional visualization, reduced instrument tremors, and increased instrument flexibility. These systems can be performed via a single umbilical incision or through multiport methods, offering a range of options to suit different procedures [42].

Artificial Intelligence (AI) algorithms and Augmented Reality (AR) overlays are emerging technologies that hold immense potential to revolutionize surgical practice. These technologies offer real-time assistance to surgeons, analyzing vast amounts of data to enhance anatomical recognition and surgical decision-making. AR overlays integrate digital information into the surgeon's view of the patient, offering intuitive visual guidance and improving spatial awareness. This technology allows surgeons to navigate complex anatomies more effectively and confidently perform procedures. While still in the early stages of adoption, AI and AR hold promise for not just improving but optimizing surgical outcomes [43, 44].

3.11 Overall insights into these updates

Laparoscopic cholecystectomy (LC) has revolutionized the surgical treatment of benign GB diseases following conventional cholecystectomy. However, there needs to be a clear consensus on the superiority of standard LC versus modified LC methods. While some studies suggest specific advantages of modified techniques, unanimity still needs to be discovered. The paramount importance of patient safety cannot be ignored. The principles of safe cholecystectomy must not be compromised when choosing a surgical method. With its rigorous adherence to the CVS, the standard LC procedure remains the foundational approach. While modified techniques offer potential benefits, the debate about their overall superiority continues, necessitating a balanced approach that prioritizes patient safety. Ensuring that improved cosmetic results do not undermine safety underscores the importance of experienced surgeons and careful patient selection when considering modified LC methods [18].

Safety issues: Early complications following LC include bile duct injury (BDI), bile duct leak, SSI, and intra-abdominal infection. BDI is particularly critical, although its incidence has decreased to an estimated 0.4–1.5% as surgeons' skills have advanced [18]. A recent meta-analysis highlighted lower complication rates with three-port and standard LC methods [45]. Another meta-analysis indicated comparable rates of early postoperative complications across methods, with needlescopic LC showing a lower incidence of SSI [46]. No significant differences in complications were found between robot-assisted and LC [47].

Surgery time: Procedure duration varies across techniques. Three-port techniques have shorter surgery times than standard LC [48]. Single-incision LC and needlescopic cholecystectomy have also been associated with shorter times than standard LC [46]. However, robot-assisted cholecystectomy requires a longer duration [47].

Postoperative pain: Modified LC techniques often demonstrate advantages in postoperative pain. Single-incision robot-assisted cholecystectomy has been reported to yield the least postoperative pain, followed by other single-incision approaches [45]. Needlescopic LC also shows promise in minimizing postoperative pain [46]. Conversely, meta-analyses comparing single-incision LC with multiport methods have not consistently shown differences in pain [48].

Length of hospital stay is another crucial consideration in LC outcomes. Studies have indicated shorter hospital stays with three-port LC compared to standard LC and single-incision robot-assisted and needlescopic techniques [45, 46]. However, these findings generally do not account for emergency surgeries, such as those for acute cholecystitis, which typically require more extended hospital stays regardless of the surgical method [18].

4. Special situations in laparoscopic cholecystectomy

Laparoscopic cholecystectomy (LC) can present unique challenges in specific clinical situations. The term "difficult GB" implies that the procedure may be complex and risky, posing potential complications for the patient. While there is no precise definition of "difficult GB," it generally refers to a cholecystectomy that is likely to be more complex than a conventional one. Most papers indicate acute or chronic inflammation owing to cholecystitis as a cause of surgical complications. However, other factors such as previous cholecystostomy, liver cirrhosis, coagulation therapy or abnormalities, and previous upper abdominal surgery are mentioned elsewhere. Although the incidence of difficult GBs varies by series, it is believed that one in every six GBs is "difficult." By understanding and preparing for these specific clinical situations, surgeons can optimize outcomes and reduce the risks associated with LC [49, 50].

4.1 Cholecysto-choledocho-lithiasis

Several strategies exist to treat patients with cholecystolithiasis and bile duct stones. The most applied method involves clearance of the bile ducts by endoscopic sphincterotomy, followed by LC. A sizable population-based analysis in British Columbia showed that 44.4% of cases followed an early cholecystectomy strategy within two days after sphincterotomy, while 55.6% opted for delayed cholecystectomy. This variation reflects clinical practice, where scheduling can differ widely. Some studies have noted higher conversion rates compared to standard LC. However, overall conversion rates for early LC after sphincterotomy are generally lower

(4–23% for early vs. 8–55% for delayed), and early cholecystectomy results in fewer recurrent biliary events (2–10% early vs. 24–47% delayed) [49, 51]. An RCT comparing LC within three days to 6–8 weeks post-sphincterotomy found no significant differences in conversion rates (4.3% early vs. 8.7% delayed), operating times, or hospital stays, but noted a substantial difference in biliary events during the waiting period (2% early vs. 36.2% delayed). This study's findings are crucial, leading to the ESGE guidelines strongly recommending performing LC within two weeks of endoscopic sphincterotomy based on moderate-quality evidence [52].

Preoperative imaging is crucial for identifying CBD stones before LC. Techniques such as EUS and MRCP are highly effective in detecting these stones. EUS provides detailed images of the biliary and pancreatic ducts, making it particularly useful for patients at high risk of CBD stones. MRCP, on the other hand, offers a non-invasive alternative with high sensitivity and specificity, allowing for accurate diagnosis. Implementing these imaging modalities in the preoperative phase helps plan the appropriate surgical approach and reduces the risk of complications during surgery. *Intraoperative cholangiography* is a valuable technique for confirming the presence of CBD stones during LC. This procedure involves the injection of a contrast dye into the biliary system, followed by X-ray imaging to visualize the ducts. If stones are detected, surgeons can proceed with intraoperative endoscopic retrograde cholangiopancreatography (ERCP) or laparoscopic CBD exploration to remove the stones. This ensures the complete clearance of stones and minimizes the risk of postoperative complications. By incorporating intraoperative cholangiography, surgeons can make real-time decisions that improve patient outcomes and reduce the need for additional procedures. *Postoperative ERCP* is a critical intervention for patients who are found to have CBD stones after LC. ERCP combines endoscopy and fluoroscopy to diagnose and treat conditions of the biliary or pancreatic ductal systems. If stones are identified postoperatively, ERCP can be employed to extract them, thereby alleviating symptoms and preventing complications such as cholangitis or pancreatitis. This procedure is especially beneficial for patients who develop symptoms indicative of retained stones, ensuring that they receive prompt and effective treatment [52–54].

4.2 Mirizzi syndrome

Mirizzi syndrome, also known as extrinsic bile compression syndrome, is a rare complication of cholecystitis and chronic cholelithiasis. It occurs due to the obliteration of the GB infundibulum or cystic duct by the impaction of one or more gallstones in these anatomical structures. This leads to the compression of the adjacent bile duct, resulting in partial or complete obstruction of the common hepatic duct and triggering liver dysfunction. ERCP, our most accurate diagnostic tool, plays a crucial role in identifying this condition. Intraoperative cholangiography helps delineate the anatomy and avoid bile duct injuries. Traditionally, surgical treatment involves an incision at the bottom of the GB and stone removal. If fistulas are present, a partial cholecystectomy is performed; alternatively, a cholecysto-choledocho-duodenostomy can be considered. Endoscopic treatment options include biliary drainage and stone extraction. While many surgeons believe that LC is contraindicated in Mirizzi syndrome due to the presence of inflammatory tissue and adhesions in Calot's triangle, others argue that, with the right skills and equipment, the laparoscopic approach is feasible and safe, particularly for Mirizzi syndrome type I and II. Despite its technical challenges, LC for Mirizzi syndrome is becoming increasingly accepted (**Figure 6**) [55, 56].

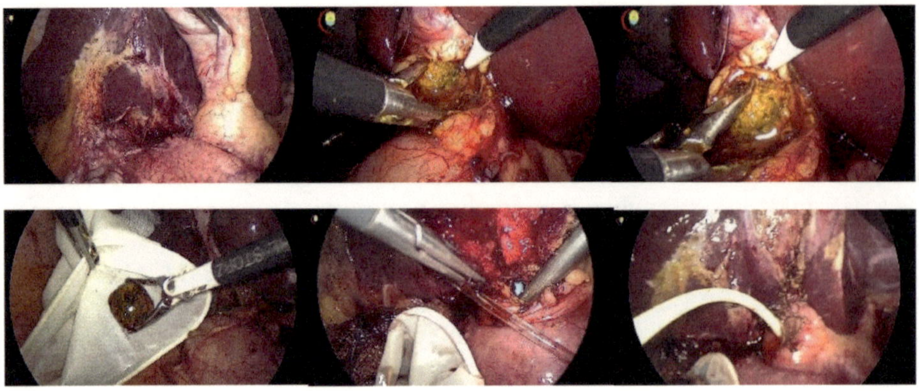

Figure 6.
Mirizzi syndrome management.

4.3 Cystic duct stones

Cystic duct stones pose significant risks during LC, including intractable pain, Mirizzi syndrome, and postoperative GB issues. Their incidence is attributed to the complex cystic duct anatomy, surgical techniques, and surgeon expertise. Reports indicate a residual stone rate of approximately 12.3% after LC, likely increasing with higher procedure volumes globally. The "semicut" technique (**Figure** 7), recently introduced for LC, modifies clamping sequences and incisions in the cystic duct to enhance stone removal and minimize complications.

This approach, compatible with existing surgical practices, aims to effectively prevent residual stones and associated postoperative symptoms. It maintains operational efficiency without compromising duct integrity, potentially improving patient outcomes by reducing complications related to retained cystic duct stones. Ongoing monitoring will assess its long-term efficacy in preventing postoperative discomfort [57].

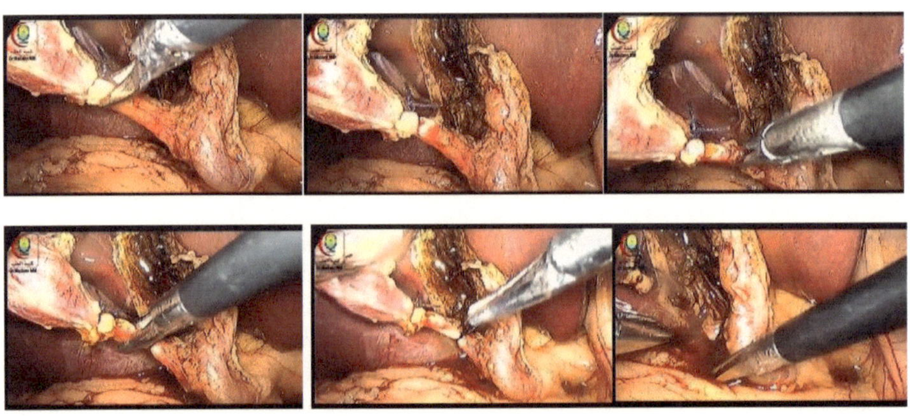

Figure 7.
Semicut technique is possible and safe with the use of Madany triangle, even in the presence of a caterpillar hump of the tight hepatic artery.

4.4 Mucocele of the GB

Mucocele of the GB, characterized by distension and dilation due to chronic accumulation of sterile, non-pigmented mucus, is often discovered incidentally during surgery. It primarily results from chronic cystic duct obstruction by impacted stones, frequently associated with gallstone disease. The preferred treatment, LC, with open cholecystectomy reserved for significantly distended or thick-walled GBs, has shown promising results in improving patient outcomes. Intraoperative aspiration of the GB's mucoid contents is crucial, facilitating easier grasping and manipulation and reducing the risk of rupture and spillage. Preoperative management includes hydration and broad-spectrum antibiotics, with cholecystectomy recommended during the same hospital admission. Recent studies highlight the importance of intraoperative aspiration, showing lower morbidity, shorter hospital stays, and fewer complications compared to non-aspiration cases. Routine preoperative ultrasound or CT scans help in planning the procedure. Given these findings, mandatory aspiration of mucocele contents during LC is now recommended, a practice that has significantly contributed to the positive outcomes of our patients [58].

4.5 Acute cholecystitis

Acute cholecystitis (**Figure 8**) management has long debated the timing of cholecystectomy, with early versus delayed approaches scrutinized despite the advent of laparoscopic techniques. Recent evidence strongly supports early cholecystectomy as superior, demonstrating lower morbidity, shorter hospital stays, and reduced hospitalization costs without significant differences in conversion rates [50]. The Tokyo guidelines define early cholecystectomy typically within 72 hours from onset but acknowledge challenges in precise timing, spanning definitions from admission within 24 hours to up to 1 week, while delayed cholecystectomy is generally after six weeks. Updated in 2018, these guidelines categorize acute cholecystitis by severity, guiding management strategies based on inflammatory status and organ dysfunction. For moderate cases (grade II), early LC is recommended for low-risk patients in experienced centers. At the same time, severe cases (grade III) may also benefit from early intervention under intensive care and expert surgical management. In cases where early cholecystectomy poses high risks, urgent GB drainage is preferred for source control, ideally in specialized centers with high procedural volumes. Time sensitivity in acute cholecystitis surgery is underscored by findings from the Swedish GallRiks Registry, indicating increased bile duct injury rates with delayed surgery [50, 59, 60].

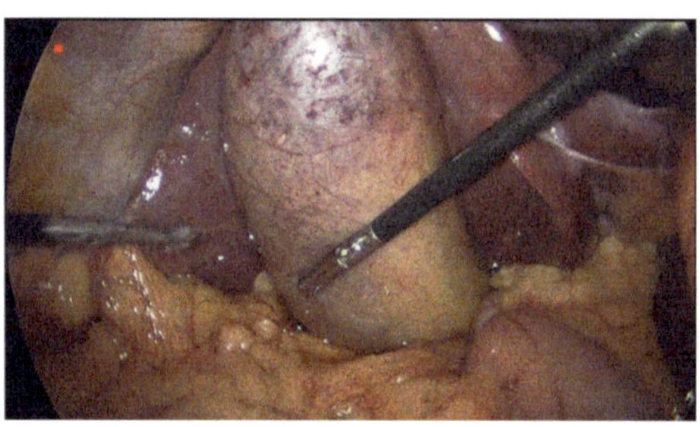

Figure 8.
Acute cholecystitis.

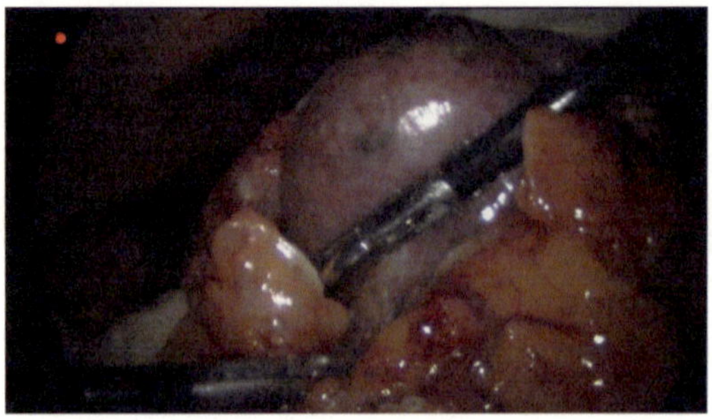

Figure 9.
Perforated GB.

4.6 Perforated gallbladder

Perforated GB (**Figure 9**) presents a critical surgical scenario necessitating immediate intervention to prevent sepsis. Emergency surgery is imperative, aiming to remove the source of infection and achieve adequate drainage. Preoperative administration of broad-spectrum antibiotics is crucial to mitigate systemic infection risks and optimize surgical outcomes. In cases of extensive inflammation or necrosis, the consideration of subtotal cholecystectomy is not just a suggestion; it is a potential game-changer. This procedure can effectively manage compromised tissue, reducing the risk of bile leakage or further infection. Cholecystostomy may be used in some instances [61–63].

4.7 Short or absent cystic duct

Intraoperative cholangiography is essential for accurate identification of the biliary anatomy, reducing the risk of bile duct injuries during LC. The fundus-first technique, which involves dissecting from the GB fundus down to the neck, can be beneficial in identifying the cystic duct, especially in challenging cases. However, in instances of severe anatomical difficulties, conversion to open surgery may be necessary to ensure patient safety and a successful outcome (**Figures 10** and **11**) [20, 52].

4.8 Seatbelt effect of the cystic artery and its branches on the gallbladder

The seatbelt effect of the cystic artery and its branches on the GB presents a significant challenge during LC. The key to managing this situation lies in meticulous dissection around the cystic artery using advanced energy devices to prevent bleeding and ensure a clear operative field. Achieving the CVS is crucial in this context to avoid injury to the bile ducts and vessels, providing a safer approach and reducing the risk of complications. By combining careful dissection techniques with the principle of CVS, surgeons can effectively manage the anatomical complexities posed by the cystic artery and its branches (**Figure 3**) [30, 31].

4.9 Frozen Calot's triangle and retrograde cholecystectomy

In cases of frozen Calot's triangle encountered during LC, effective management strategies are essential to navigate through the challenging anatomy. Advanced imaging techniques play a crucial role in preoperative planning, allowing surgeons to assess

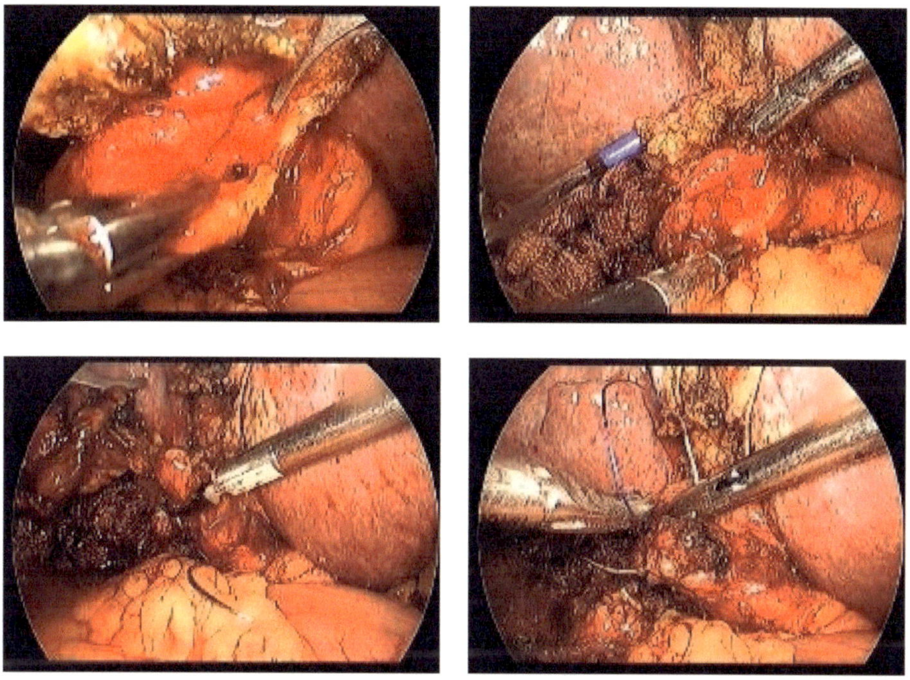

Figure 10.
Laparoscopic management of an absent cystic duct (the GB open directly in the CBD).

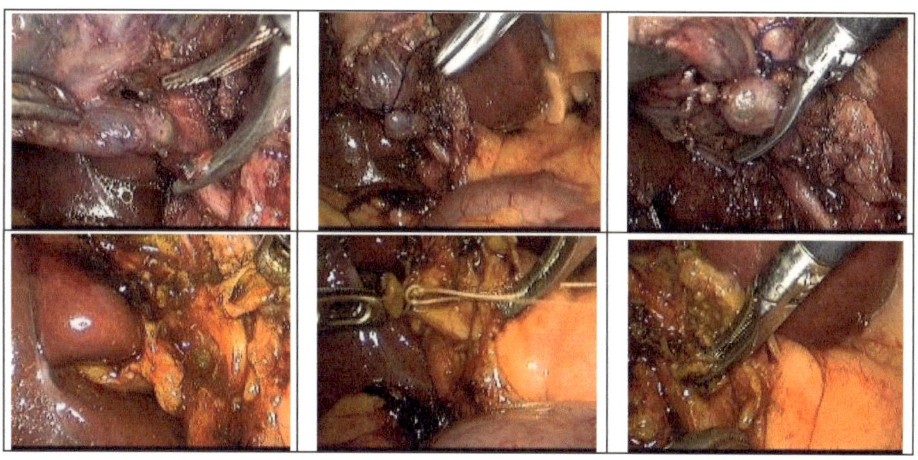

Figure 11.
Laparoscopic management of an absent cystic duct (the GB opens directly in the right hepatic duct).

the extent of inflammation and fibrosis surrounding Calot's triangle. This helps in strategizing the approach for dissection [64–66].

Retrograde (Fundus-first) approach (**Figure 12**) is a specialized technique of dissecting the GB from the liver bed utilized in cases presenting challenges such as severe inflammation or complex anatomical variations. By initiating dissection from the fundus of the GB toward the cystic duct, surgeons can navigate around potentially obstructive structures or areas of high inflammation more effectively. This method

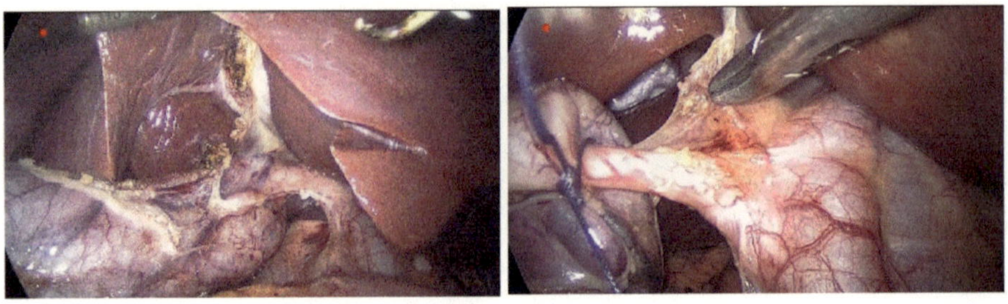

Figure 12.
Fundus-first approach.

allows for better visualization and maneuverability in difficult surgical scenarios, reducing the risk of inadvertent injury and improving overall surgical outcomes [67, 68]. It is often employed in cases with frozen Calot's triangle, initiating dissection at the GB fundus, and carefully progressing toward Calot's triangle. This method aids in gradually freeing up adhesions and identifying critical structures amidst the inflammatory changes [64–66].

In severe instances where dissection is exceedingly difficult or risky, *subtotal cholecystectomy* (fenestrating or reconstituting type) may be considered. This involves leaving a portion of the GB attached to mitigate the risk of bile duct injury while managing the frozen triangle effectively. The left GB portion must undergo mucosal ablation with diathermy to abolish its secretory function. By integrating these techniques, surgeons can navigate the complexities of frozen Calot's triangle more safely and effectively during LC [64–66]. In old age, high-risk patients with frozen Calot's triangle, we may reserve to just open the fundus, remove the stones, and then insert a drain inside the GB *(cholecystolithotomy)* [64–66].

4.10 Intrahepatic gallbladder

In cases of intrahepatic GB (**Figure 13**), preoperative imaging plays a pivotal role by precisely delineating the GB's position within the liver and its relationship with adjacent liver tissue. This imaging allows surgeons to plan a meticulous approach to dissection, aimed at avoiding inadvertent liver injury. The modified technique

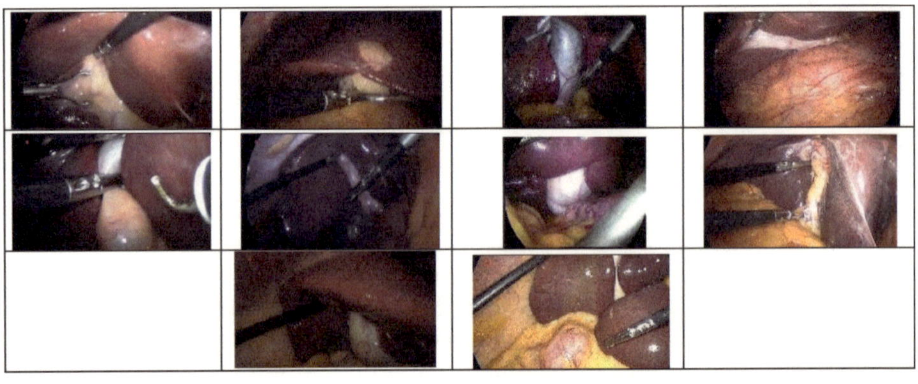

Figure 13.
Partial intrahepatic GB.

involves careful dissection around the GB, ensuring preservation of hepatic parenchyma and minimizing the risk of complications. In more complex scenarios, partial hepatectomy may be necessary to safely remove the intrahepatic GB [69, 70].

4.11 Cholecystostomy

Percutaneous cholecystostomy (PC) is utilized due to its efficacy in managing acute cholecystitis in high-risk or critically ill patients. This approach involves inserting a catheter directly into the GB under ultrasound or CT guidance to drain infected bile and alleviate symptoms like pain and fever, stabilizing patients before considering definitive surgery. Indications for PC include severe systemic illness, GB perforation, or a bridging therapy to surgical intervention. Improved imaging guidance ensures precise catheter placement, minimizing risks such as inadvertent organ puncture. Catheter design innovations aim to reduce dislodgement and infection rates, while adjunctive therapies like intracholecystic thrombolytics are explored to aid bile drainage and hasten inflammation resolution, especially in cases of malignancy [71].

4.12 Subtotal cholecystectomy

Subtotal cholecystectomy is used when LC becomes challenging due to factors like severe inflammation or difficult anatomical conditions, preventing a CVS. It involves partial removal of the GB, leaving either an open (fenestrating) or closed (reconstituting) remnant to minimize the risk of common bile duct injuries and other complications. This approach, with an incidence ranging from 4.00% to 9.38%, despite addressing complexities in GB surgery, it poses risks such as biliary fistulae and retained stones. Skillful execution is crucial to prevent complications like bile leakage and remnant GB cholecystitis. Despite its immediate benefits, ongoing research is needed to explore alternative techniques and assess long-term risks, including potential malignancy in residual GB tissue, ensuring optimal safety and efficacy in difficult surgical contexts [72].

4.13 Completion cholecystectomy

Laparoscopic completion cholecystectomy (LCC) addresses symptomatic residual GB or cystic duct stump stones left after an initial cholecystectomy. Residual GB remnants can harbor or develop stones, causing recurrent symptoms. Post-cholecystectomy syndrome (PCS) occurs in 10–40% of patients. Diagnosis relies on clinical suspicion and imaging such as ultrasonography, MRCP, ERCP, and EUS. LCC has shown good results with experienced surgeons. LCC had a low conversion rate to open surgery (8.3%). LCC is safe and effective, offering a solution for symptomatic GB residuals and improving patient outcomes [73].

4.14 Repeat cholecystectomy

Repeat cholecystectomy (RC) is often necessary when patients develop symptoms after an initial cholecystectomy, which is commonly owing to undiagnosed GB duplication. This congenital condition is difficult to diagnose, particularly when preoperative imaging such as ultrasound or CT scans fail to detect it, which happens in less than half of instances. When GB duplication is suspected, an intraoperative cholangiogram is recommended, especially if scarring or patient habitus obscures the inferior liver margin. Recognizing this aberration is critical for avoiding inadequate surgical care, reducing perioperative difficulties, and minimizing long-term patient morbidity [74].

4.15 Conversion cholecystectomy

The rate of conversion from laparoscopic to open cholecystectomy varies widely depending on clinical presentations, surgeon experience, and the pathology encountered. A large prospective study across the UK, analyzing 5738 LCs performed by a single surgeon over 28 years, showed that 28 patients (0.49%) required conversion to open cholecystectomy, with a morbidity rate of 33%. The main reasons for conversion were dense adhesions (32%) and impacted bile duct stones (25%). Additionally, 173 patients (3%) underwent fundus first cholecystectomy (FFC) with a 17.3% morbidity rate, and 6 patients (0.1%) had subtotal cholecystectomy with no complications. These techniques reduced the potential conversion rate from 3.5% to 0.49%. While open conversion carries high morbidity and should be a last resort, subspecialization, and high emergency case volume, along with FFC and subtotal cholecystectomy, effectively lower conversion rates and associated complications in challenging cholecystectomies. Open conversion, while sometimes necessary for patient safety, should not be viewed as a failure but as a safe option during complex cases [75].

4.16 Adhesiolysis with laparoscopic cholecystectomy

Adhesiolysis is a critical aspect of LC when encountering extensive adhesions, necessitating careful dissection techniques using advanced energy devices to safely separate adhesions without causing injury. This meticulous approach ensures that vital structures are preserved while navigating through adherent tissues. However, it is important to anticipate extended operating times due to the intricacies involved in adhesiolysis, which can prolong surgical duration compared to standard LC procedures. Surgeons must be prepared for these challenges to effectively manage adhesions during LC, ensuring patient safety and optimal surgical outcomes [76].

4.17 Ventral hernia with laparoscopic cholecystectomy

Concurrent repair of ventral hernia during LC allows for efficient management of both conditions within the same surgical session, optimizing patient recovery and reducing overall healthcare costs. Surgeons may opt to use mesh placement to reinforce the hernia repair and prevent recurrence. Preoperative planning plays a crucial role, involving detailed assessment and decision-making regarding trocar placement and access points to ensure optimal outcomes for both the hernia repair and cholecystectomy. Prospective studies with additional procedural-specific information for hernia repairs and cholecystectomy are required; nonetheless, in cholecystectomy patients who do not show evidence of acute infection, it is likely safe to conduct both procedures concurrently [77].

4.18 Cirrhotic liver

Preoperative optimization in cirrhotic patients undergoing cholecystectomy involves optimizing liver function and managing coagulopathy to mitigate

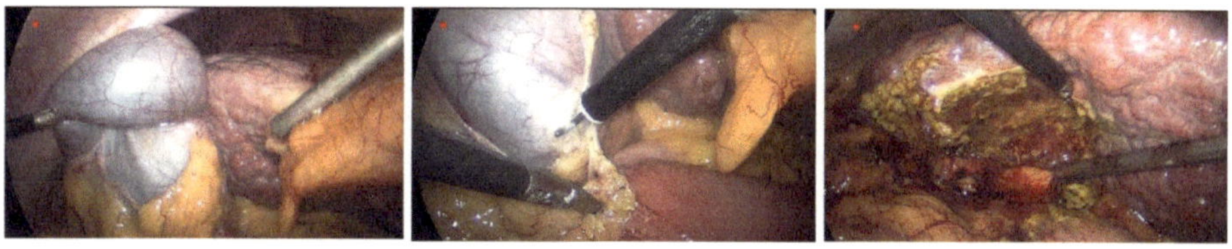

Figure 14.
Meticulous dissection is essential during LC in patients with cirrhotic liver.

perioperative risks. Utilizing a low-pressure pneumoperitoneum strategy is crucial as it helps minimize the risk of bleeding and hemodynamic instability. Meticulous dissection techniques should be employed to handle liver tissue delicately and reduce intraoperative bleeding [78] (**Figure 14**). Patients with cirrhosis had a higher incidence of postoperative complications compared to non-cirrhotic patients. However, cholecystectomy should not be delayed when clinically indicated. Perioperative mortality significantly increased with higher Child-Pugh class, MELD score, and acuity [79].

4.19 Morbid obesity

Morbid obesity is widely recognized as a significant risk factor contributing to the complexity of cholecystectomy. A recent review examining factors associated with the conversion from laparoscopic to open surgery highlighted that 8 out of 19 studies specifically identified a higher conversion rate among patients with a BMI exceeding 30 kg/m^2. This increased conversion rate is attributed to technical challenges such as the length and positioning of trocars, adipose infiltration of Calot's triangle, and difficulties in visualizing anatomical structures. However, the extent to which obesity alone directly causes surgical complexity remains uncertain [50]. In a recent approach, Russell and Aroori emphasize several key strategies to enhance safety and efficacy. Following pneumoperitoneum establishment through a supra-umbilical incision, they advocate for placing a fascial suture to ensure secure closure, thereby reducing the likelihood of incisional hernias and inadvertent bowel injuries. Prior to port placement, they reposition the patient on the operating table to achieve an ergonomic setup. Alongside standard ports, they incorporate an additional twelve-millimeter port in the left upper quadrant. This port accommodates a fan retractor, facilitating gentle retraction of the duodenum inferiorly. This maneuver enhances exposure for meticulous dissection of Calot's triangle and potentially mitigates the risk of injuring a fatty liver [80].

4.20 When is it necessary to put a drain?

The use of surgical drainage after LC remains debated despite its widespread use. Advocates argue it prevents complications like postoperative collections and aids $CO2$ release, potentially reducing shoulder pain and peritoneal irritation. Drawbacks include risks of vascular or intestinal injury, infections related to the drain, and omental blockage. Also, it is annoying the patient. Absence of bile or blood in the drain does not ensure the absence of complications. Recent guidelines discourage routine drainage after uncomplicated elective cholecystectomy. In acute cholecystitis, guidelines are unclear, leaving drainage decisions to the surgeon discretion [49, 81, 82].

4.21 Post-cholecystectomy syndrome

Post-cholecystectomy syndrome (PCS) encompasses a range of symptoms like right upper quadrant abdominal pain, dyspepsia, and jaundice that occur after cholecystectomy. The syndrome can manifest early or late post-surgery and affects a substantial number of patients, with reported incidences varying up to 40%, higher in females. Causes of PCS are categorized into extra-biliary factors such as reflux esophagitis, peptic ulcer disease, and irritable bowel syndrome, and biliary factors including biliary duct injury, retained stones, bile salt-induced diarrhea, bile duct strictures, recurrent stones, or sphincter of Oddi dysfunction. Diagnosis relies on clinical presentation, supported by laboratory tests and imaging. Management strategies for biliary causes include ERCP for stone removal, sphincterotomy for sphincter of Oddi dysfunction, or surgical correction for bile duct strictures. Extra-biliary causes are managed through medical therapies targeting specific conditions [83].

5. Conclusion

In conclusion, this chapter has traced the progression from the classic approach of LC to recent advancements, emphasizing innovations in visualization, instrumentation, and surgical techniques that have further improved safety and efficacy. Key updates include strategies for reducing complications, managing complex cases, and utilizing enhanced imaging tools that offer greater precision. As the field progresses, ongoing technological developments continue to improve LC. Future directions may involve broader applications of robotic assistance, artificial intelligence for intraoperative decision-making, and minimally invasive techniques that further decrease the surgical impact.

Declaration statements

The author acknowledges the usage of Grammarly AI tool for language polishing of the manuscript.

Author details

Mohie El-Din Mostafa Madany
Aswan University, Aswan, Egypt

*Address all correspondence to: mohie25@yahoo.com;
mohie.madany@med.aswu.edu.eg

References

[1] Majumder A, Altieri MS, Brunt LM. How do I do it: Laparoscopic cholecystectomy. Annals of Laparoscopic and Endoscopic Surgery. 2020;**5**:15-19. Available from: https://ales.amegroups.org/article/view/5766 [Accessed: June 11, 2024]

[2] Hassler KR, Collins JT, Philip K, Jones MW. Laparoscopic cholecystectomy. In: StatPearls. Treasure Island (FL): StatPearls Publishing; 2024. Available from: http://www.ncbi.nlm.nih.gov/books/NBK448145/ [Accessed: June 11, 2024]

[3] Grüter AAJ, Daams F, Bonjer HJ, van Duijvendijk P, Tuynman JB. Video-based surgical quality assessment collaborators. Surgical quality assessment of critical view of safety in 283 laparoscopic cholecystectomy videos by surgical residents and surgeons. Surgical Endoscopy. Jul 2024;**38**(7):3609-3614

[4] Strasberg SM, Brunt LM. Rationale and use of the critical view of safety in laparoscopic cholecystectomy. Journal of the American College of Surgeons. 2010;**211**(1):132-138

[5] Iseda N, Iguchi T, Itoh S, Sasaki S, Honboh T, Yoshizumi T, et al. Textbook outcome in the laparoscopic cholecystectomy of acute cholecystitis. Asian Journal of Endoscopic Surgery. 2023;**16**(4):741-746

[6] Gavriilidis P, Catena F, de Angelis G, de Angelis N. Consequences of the spilled gallstones during laparoscopic cholecystectomy: A systematic review. World Journal of Emergency Surgery : WJES. 2022;**17**(1):57

[7] Marks JM, Phillips MS, Tacchino R, Roberts K, Onders R, DeNoto G, et al. Single-incision laparoscopic cholecystectomy is associated with improved cosmesis scoring at the cost of significantly higher hernia rates: 1-year results of a prospective randomized, multicenter, single-blinded trial of traditional multiport laparoscopic cholecystectomy vs single-incision laparoscopic cholecystectomy. Journal of the American College of Surgeons. 2013;**216**(6):1037-1047 discussion 1047-1048

[8] Lunevicius R. Cholecystectomy: Advances and issues. Journal of Clinical Medicine. 2022;**11**(12):3534

[9] Ye F, Wu Y, Zhou C. Effect of intravenous ketamine for postoperative analgesia in patients undergoing laparoscopic cholecystectomy: A meta-analysis. Medicine (Baltimore). 2017;**96**(51):e9147

[10] Ljungqvist O, Scott M, Fearon KC. Enhanced recovery after surgery: A review. JAMA Surgery. 2017;**152**(3):292-298

[11] Mencarini L, Vestito A, Zagari RM, Montagnani M. New developments in the ultrasonography diagnosis of gallbladder diseases. Gastroenterology Insights. 2024;**15**(1):42-68

[12] Kang KA, Kwon HJ, Ham SY, Park HJ, Shin JH, Lee SR, et al. Impacts on outcomes and management of preoperative magnetic resonance cholangiopancreatography in patients scheduled for laparoscopic cholecystectomy: For whom it should be considered? Annals of Surgical Treatment and Research. 2020;**99**(4):221-229

[13] Ahmed OMT, Gad GS, Abd El-Lateef AF. Comparing different

modalities of opioid free Anesthesia for laparoscopic cholecystectomy. SVU-International Journal of Medical Sciences. 2024;**7**(1):919-938

[14] Mohamed AH, Mohamed SR, Farouk MA. Analgesic effect of ultrasound guided regional block in laparoscopic cholecystectomy. Minia Journal of Medical Research. 2020;**31**(2):150-161

[15] Polese L, Giugliano E, Valmasoni M. Patient position in operative endoscopy. Journal of Clinical Medicine. 2023;**12**(21):6822

[16] Bessa SS, Katri KM, Talaat Korayem IM, Mahrous Badr MF. Optical trocar versus blind intial trocar insertion during laparoscopic cholecystectomy: A randomized comparative study. Alexmed Eposters. 2022;**4**(4):12-13

[17] Özdemir-van Brunschot DMD, van Laarhoven KCJHM, Scheffer GJ, Pouwels S, Wever KE, Warlé MC. What is the evidence for the use of low-pressure pneumoperitoneum? A systematic review. Surgical Endoscopy. 2016;**30**:2049-2065

[18] Sevik H, Karsidag T, Tatar C. A narrative review of technical developments for the laparoscopic cholecystectomy. Annals of Laparoscopic and Endoscopic Surgery. 2024;**9**:14-23. Available from: https://ales.amegroups.org/article/view/9918 [Accessed: June 12, 2024]

[19] Erdoğan E, Dursun A, Güler M. Safe and aesthetic; laparoscopic cholecystectomy on the bikini line. Van Health Sciences Journal. 2023;**16**(1):9-13

[20] Gupta V, Jain G. Safe laparoscopic cholecystectomy: Adoption of universal culture of safety in cholecystectomy. World Journal of Gastrointestinal Surgery. 2019;**11**(2):62-84

[21] Nip L, Tong KS, Borg CM. Three-port versus four-port technique for laparoscopic cholecystectomy: Systematic review and meta-analysis. BJS Open. 2022;**6**(2):zrac013

[22] Chatterjee A, Kumar R, Chattoraj A. Three-port laparoscopic cholecystectomy as a safe and feasible alternative to the conventional four-port laparoscopic cholecystectomy. Cureus. 2024;**16**(1):e52196

[23] Taha M, Sallam AN, Zakaria HM, Nassar A. Modified technique for two ports laparoscopic cholecystectomy: Combined safety and economic value. The Egyptian Journal of Surgery. 2019;**38**(3):511

[24] Ishikawa M, Asanoma M, Tashiro Y, Takechi H, Matsuyama K, Miyauchi T. Gasless single-port laparoscopic cholecystectomy. The Journal of Minimally Invasive Surgery. 2021;**24**(3):152-157

[25] Yang E, Nie D, Li Z. Comparison of major clinical outcomes between transvaginal NOTES and traditional laparoscopic surgery: A systematic review and meta-analysis. The Journal of Surgical Research. 2019;**244**:278-290. Available from: https://pubmed.ncbi.nlm.nih.gov/31302326/ [Accessed: June 13, 2024]

[26] Komine O, Suzuki H, Watanabe M, Nomura S, Mizutani S, Yoshino M, et al. Single-incision laparoscopic cholecystectomy with an additional needle grasper: A novel technique. Journal of Nippon Medical School. 2015;**82**(1):43-49

[27] Dip F, Lo Menzo E, White KP, Rosenthal RJ. Does near-infrared fluorescent cholangiography with indocyanine green reduce bile duct injuries and conversions to open

surgery during laparoscopic or robotic cholecystectomy?- a meta-analysis. Surgery. 2021;**169**(4):859-867

[28] Ortenzi M, Agresta F, Vettoretto N, Gerardi C, Allocati E, Botteri E, et al. Use of high energy devices (HEDs) versus electrocautery for laparoscopic cholecystectomy: A systematic review and meta-analysis of randomised controlled trials. Surgical Endoscopy. 2023;**37**(6):4249-4269

[29] Madany MEDM, Kabbash MM, Abdallah HA. Safety and feasibility of cystic artery control with bipolar electrocauterization during laparoscopic cholecystectomy. The Egyptian Journal of Surgery. 2024;**43**(2):356

[30] Jin Y, Liu R, Chen Y, Liu J, Zhao Y, Wei A, et al. Critical view of safety in laparoscopic cholecystectomy: A prospective investigation from both cognitive and executive aspects. Frontiers in Surgery. 2022;**9**:946917

[31] Madany MEDM, Soliman A, Sabra TA, Takrouney MH, Fathy M, Abdelmohsen SM. Madany triangle: A new era of laparoscopic cholecystectomy. International Journal of Surgery Open. 2024;**62**(2):144

[32] Kassem MI, Hassouna EM. Short-term outcome of total clipless laparoscopic cholecystectomy for complicated gallbladder stones in cirrhotic patients. ANZ Journal of Surgery. 2018;**88**(3):E152-E156

[33] Pereira C, Gururaj S, Varghese B. Harmonic scalpel versus clips for ligation of cystic duct in laparoscopic cholecystectomy: A systematic review. Cureus. 2022;**14**(12):e32335

[34] Madany MEDM, Kabbash MM, Mostafa HA, Maghraby AM, Ahmed MS. Safety and feasibility of cystic duct control with suture ligation during laparoscopic cholecystectomy. The Egyptian Journal of Surgery. 2024;**43**(2):579

[35] Mohamed HK, Albendary M, Wuheb AA, Ali O, Mohammed MJ, Osman M, et al. A systematic review and meta-analysis of bag extraction versus direct extraction for retrieval of gallbladder after laparoscopic cholecystectomy. Cureus. 2023;**15**(2):e35493

[36] Madany MEDM, Abd El Raheim YMS, Saad MR. Gall bladder retrieval in laparoscopic cholecystectomy. Aswan University Medical Journal. 2024;**4**(2):28-36

[37] Madany MEDM, Zakaria A, Abdelaal AH, Ahmed H, Bakr MA, Elsaid M, et al. Nasr fascial closure: a novel device for fascial closure in laparoscopic surgery. The Egyptian Journal of Surgery. 2024;**43**(1):82

[38] Madany MEDM, Zakaria A, Abdelaal AH, Ahmed H, Bakr MA, Elsaid M, et al. Madany closure: A novel technique for fascial closure in laparoscopic surgery. The Egyptian Journal of Surgery. 2024;**43**(1):116

[39] Fernandez LC, Toriz A, Hernandez J, Sanchez N, Linares E, Zenteno M, et al. Knotless choledochorraphy with barbed suture, safe and feasible. Surgical Endoscopy. 2016;**30**(8):3630-3635

[40] Martins TP, Souza DM, Souza DM. Use of multimodal anesthesia in the treatment of postoperative pain. BrJP. 2023;**6**:427-434

[41] Kaye AD, Urman RD, Rappaport Y, Siddaiah H, Cornett EM, Belani K, et al. Multimodal analgesia as an essential part of enhanced recovery protocols in the ambulatory settings. Journal of

Anaesthesiology Clinical Pharmacology. 2019;**35**(Suppl 1):S40-S45

[42] Lee EK, Park E, Oh WO, Shin NM. Comparison of the outcomes of robotic cholecystectomy and laparoscopic cholecystectomy. Annals of Surgical Treatment and Research. 2017;**93**(1):27-34

[43] Brockmeyer P, Wiechens B, Schliephake H. The role of augmented reality in the advancement of minimally invasive surgery procedures: A scoping review. Bioengineering. 2023;**10**(4):501

[44] Reza T, Bokhari SFH. Partnering with technology: Advancing laparoscopy with artificial intelligence and machine learning. Cureus. 2024;**16**(3):e56076

[45] Lin H, Zhang J, Li X, Li Y, Su S. Comparative outcomes of single-incision laparoscopic, mini-laparoscopic, four-port laparoscopic, three-port laparoscopic, and single-incision robotic cholecystectomy: A systematic review and network meta-analysis. Updates in Surgery. 2023;**75**(1):41-51

[46] Zhao JJ, Syn NL, Chong C, Tan HL, Ng JYX, Yap A, et al. Comparative outcomes of needlescopic, single-incision laparoscopic, standard laparoscopic, mini-laparotomy, and open cholecystectomy: A systematic review and network meta-analysis of 96 randomized controlled trials with 11,083 patients. Surgery. 2021;**170**(4):994-1003

[47] Han C, Shan X, Yao L, Yan P, Li M, Hu L, et al. Robotic-assisted versus laparoscopic cholecystectomy for benign gallbladder diseases: A systematic review and meta-analysis. Surgical Endoscopy. 2018;**32**(11):4377-4392

[48] Lyu Y, Cheng Y, Wang B, Zhao S, Chen L. Single-incision versus conventional multiport laparoscopic cholecystectomy: A current meta-analysis of randomized controlled trials. Surgical Endoscopy. 2020;**34**(10):4315-4329

[49] Missori G, Serra F, Gelmini R. A narrative review about difficult laparoscopic cholecystectomy: Technical tips. Laparoscopic Surgery. 2022;**6**:24-33. Available from: https://ls.amegroups.org/article/view/7535 [Accessed: June 14, 2024]

[50] Függer R. Challenging situations in cholecystectomy and strategies to overcome them. European Surgery. 2021;**53**(3):106-113

[51] Mador BD, Nathens AB, Xiong W, Panton ONM, Hameed SM. Timing of cholecystectomy following endoscopic sphincterotomy: A population-based study. Surgical Endoscopy. 2017;**31**(7):2977-2985

[52] Manes G, Paspatis G, Aabakken L, Anderloni A, Arvanitakis M, Ah-Soune P, et al. Endoscopic management of common bile duct stones: European Society of Gastrointestinal Endoscopy (ESGE) guideline. Endoscopy. 2019;**51**(05):472-491

[53] Cianci P, Restini E. Management of cholelithiasis with choledocholithiasis: Endoscopic and surgical approaches. World Journal of Gastroenterology. 2021;**27**(28):4536-4554

[54] Gaied II, Ali MM, Shehata AM, Hassan AM. Concomitant ERCP and laparoscopic cholecystectomy for management of gallstones complicated by obstructive jaundice versus two sessions procedure comparative study, Minia university hospital experience. Minia Journal of Medical Research. 2023;**34**(1):133-142

[55] Valderrama-Treviño AI, Granados-Romero JJ, Espejel-Deloiza M,

Chernitzky-Camaño J, Mera BB, Estrada-Mata AG, et al. Updates in Mirizzi syndrome. Hepatobiliary Surgery and Nutrition. 2017;**6**(3):17078-17178

[56] Toro A, Teodoro M, Khan M, Schembari E, Di Saverio S, Catena F, et al. Subtotal cholecystectomy for difficult acute cholecystitis: How to finalize safely by laparoscopy—A systematic review. World Journal of Emergency Surgery : WJES. 2021;**16**:45

[57] Liu L, Zhao Z, Yang J. "Semicut" skill on the cystic duct in laparoscopic cholecystectomy. Frontiers in Surgery. 2023;**9**:1004290

[58] Shirah BH, Shirah HA, Albeladi KB. The value of intraoperative percutaneous aspiration of the mucocele of the gallbladder for safe laparoscopic management. Updates in Surgery. 2018;**70**(4):495-502

[59] Blohm M, Österberg J, Sandblom G, Lundell L, Hedberg M, Enochsson L. The sooner, the better? The importance of optimal timing of cholecystectomy in acute cholecystitis: Data from the National Swedish Registry for gallstone surgery, Gallriks. Journal of Gastrointestinal Surgery. 2017;**21**(1):33-40

[60] Okamoto K, Suzuki K, Takada T, Strasberg SM, Asbun HJ, Endo I, et al. Tokyo guidelines 2018: Flowchart for the management of acute cholecystitis. Journal of Hepato-Biliary-Pancreatic Sciences. 2018;**25**(1):55-72

[61] Sharma S, Trehan V, Ranjan P, Singh A. Gall bladder perforation: Critical analysis of management at tertiary care Centre. International Surgery Journal. 2023;**10**(2):235-239

[62] Warsinggih M, Arsyad A, Faruk M. Gallbladder perforation: A rare case report. International Journal of Surgery Case Reports. 2023;**104**:107927

[63] Rajput D, Gupta A, Kumar S, Singla T, Srikanth K, Chennatt J. Clinical spectrum and management outcome in gallbladder perforation-a sinister entity: Retrospective study from sub-Himalayan region of India. Turkish Journal of Surgery. 2022;**38**(1):025-035

[64] Sewefy AM, Hassanen AM, Atyia AM, Gaafar AM. Retroinfundibular laparoscopic cholecystectomy versus standard laparoscopic cholecystectomy in difficult cases. International Journal of Surgery. 2017;**43**:75-80

[65] Shinde J, Pandit S. Innovative approach to a frozen Calot's triangle during laparoscopic cholecystectomy. The Indian Journal of Surgery. 2015;**77**(6):554-557

[66] Yildirim AC, Zeren S, Ekici MF, Yaylak F, Algin MC, Arik O. Comparison of Fenestrating and reconstituting subtotal cholecystectomy techniques in difficult cholecystectomy. Cureus. 2022;**14**(2):e22441

[67] Garzali IU, Aburumman A, Alsardia Y, Alabdallat B, Wraikat S, Aloun A. Is fundus first laparoscopic cholecystectomy a better option than conventional laparoscopic cholecystectomy for difficult cholecystectomy? A systematic review and meta-analysis. Updates in Surgery. 2022;**74**(6):1797-1803

[68] Sormaz İC. Technical solutions for difficult laparoscopic cholecystectomies: Fundus-first technique and partial cholecystectomy. Ulusal Travma ve Acil Cerrahi Dergisi. 2018;**24**(1):66-70. Available from: https://www.journalagent.com/travma/pdfs/UTD-26795-CLINICAL_ARTICLE-SORMAZ.pdf [Accessed: June 13, 2024]

[69] Al-Tarakji M, AlFkey R, Aljohary H, Sameer M, Muhammad AS. Successful surgical Management of Unusual Gallbladder Anatomy through Laparoscopic Cholecystectomy of ectopic gallbladder. Cureus. 2021;**13**(11):e19884

[70] Segura-Sampedro JJ, Navarro-Sánchez A, Ashrafian H, Martínez-Isla A. Laparoscopic approach to the intrahepatic gallbladder: A case report. Revista Española de Enfermedades Digestivas. 2015;**107**(2):122-123

[71] Gulaya K, Desai SS, Sato K. Percutaneous Cholecystostomy: Evidence-based current clinical practice. Semin Intervent Radiol. 2016;**33**(4):291-296

[72] Ramírez-Giraldo C, Torres-Cuellar A, Van-Londoño I. State of the art in subtotal cholecystectomy: An overview. Frontiers in Surgery. 2023;**10**:1142579

[73] Elnabi MH, Hassan RA, Soliman HFA, Abdelgawaad MS. Laparoscopic completion cholecystectomy for patients with residual gallstone disease: A single-center experience. The Egyptian Journal of Surgery. 2023;**42**(3):635

[74] Wang TN, Shriki JE, Marquardt DL. Repeat laparoscopic cholecystectomy for duplicated gallbladder after 16-year interval. Federal Practitioner. 2022;**39**(2):e1-e5

[75] Nassar AHM, Zanati HE, Ng HJ, Khan KS, Wood C. Open conversion in laparoscopic cholecystectomy and bile duct exploration: Subspecialisation safely reduces the conversion rates. Surgical Endoscopy. 2022;**36**(1):550-558

[76] Park JH, Kim DJ, Park JH. Does laparoscopic Adhesiolysis reduce the risk of small bowel obstruction related readmissions and reoperations compared to open Adhesiolysis? The Journal of Minimally Invasive Surgery. 2020;**23**(2):86-92

[77] Becker TP, Duggan B, Rao V, Deleon G, Pei K. Outcomes of concurrent ventral hernia repair and cholecystectomy compared to ventral hernia repair alone. Cureus. 2023;**15**(9):e45699

[78] Newman KL, Johnson KM, Cornia PB, Wu P, Itani K, Ioannou GN. Perioperative evaluation and Management of Patients with cirrhosis: Risk assessment, surgical outcomes, and future directions. Clinical Gastroenterology and Hepatology. 2020;**18**(11):2398-2414.e3

[79] Gad EH, Ayoup E, Kamel Y, Zakareya T, Abbasy M, Nada A, et al. Surgical management of laparoscopic cholecystectomy (LC) related major bile duct injuries; predictors of short- and long-term outcomes in a tertiary Egyptian center-a retrospective cohort study. Annals of Medicine and Surgery. 2018;**36**:219-230

[80] Russell TB, Aroori S. How we do it: Laparoscopic cholecystectomy in patients with severe obesity. Turkish Journal of Surgery. 2021;**37**(4):413-416

[81] Pisano M, Allievi N, Gurusamy K, Borzellino G, Cimbanassi S, Boerna D, et al. 2020 world Society of Emergency Surgery updated guidelines for the diagnosis and treatment of acute calculus cholecystitis. World Journal of Emergency Surgery : WJES. 2020;**15**(1):61

[82] Yang SC, Chang KY, Wei LF, Shyr YM, Ho CM. To drain or not to drain: The association between residual intraperitoneal gas and post-laparoscopic shoulder pain for laparoscopic

cholecystectomy. Scientific Reports. 2021;**11**(1):7447

[83] Saleem S, Weissman S, Gonzalez H, Rojas PG, Inayat F, Alshati A, et al. Post-cholecystectomy syndrome: A retrospective study analysing the associated demographics, aetiology, and healthcare utilization. Translational Gastroenterology and Hepatology. 2021;**6**(0):58-64. Available from: https://tgh.amegroups.org/article/view/5792 [Accessed: June 18, 2024]